GOODBYE ALLERGIES

Goodbye Allergies

JUDGE TOM R. BLAINE

introduction by
SAM E. ROBERTS, M.D.
EMERITUS PROFESSOR OF OTOLARYNGOLOGY,
UNIVERSITY OF KANSAS MEDICAL SCHOOL

The Citadel Press   SECAUCUS, NEW JERSEY

To the medical pioneers,
living and dead,
of hypoglycemia and hypoadrenocorticism,
this book is respectfully dedicated.

Sixth paperbound printing, 1972

ISBN 0-8065-0139-1

CONTENTS

INTRODUCTION

Every person who has any type of allergy—mild or debilitating—should read this book. Every practising physician should have this book in his private library. He should read it with an open mind and be willing to give his patients the benefit of his unbiased opinion after a diagnosis of adrenal cortical insufficiency has been established by laboratory findings or by clinical observance. Hypoglycemia (low blood sugar) is nearly always present. Clinical manifestations, such as exhaustion, gastro-intestinal complaints, abdominal pain, loss of appetite, food phobias, etc. usually accompany these deficiencies.

The world stands on the threshold of the new knowledge of applied nutrition and greater knowledge of other deficiencies and imbalances. Judge Blaine has emphasized the constitutional approach to allergy—an approach which most physicians, esspecially the allergists, have failed even to recognize as a possible therapeutic tool in the management of allergy.

The reason for this failure is the fact that clinical nutrition is not taught in our medical schools. This book is a paradox in medical education, for it has the intelligent layman teaching the physician fundamental facts about nutrition. Most of the allergists I know are honest, conscientious, and dedicated men. They are still, however, practising medicine as it was taught to them. I was one of these doctors for the first twenty-five years of my professional life. At the end of this period I weighed my accomplishments and found them wanting. For months I kept a daily tabulation of all my patients' progress, and recorded my observations under four headings: (1) those really helped, (2) those for whom I did little to relieve their troubles, (3) those for whom nothing could be done with our present store of knowledge, and (4) those who were made worse by surgery. There were too many patients in the last three classifications.

Judge Blaine wisely takes into account the emphasis of the constitutional approach to various disorders and the vital character of glandular activities; and he finds, as might be expected, that various patients suffer from various inadequacies and that glandular difficulties are often closely related to dietary problems. If the patient carefully follows the recommended nutritional regime, I am certain he will not have to continue taking glandular extracts indefinitely. It is axiomatic that if the endocrine glands are supplied with adequate and congenial chemical media they will eventually secrete their own hormones.

I am tremendously impressed by the mass of knowledge Judge Blaine has gleaned from his reading on the subject of vitamin E, hypoglycemia, hypoadrenocorticism, and other glandular deficiencies and imbalances.

SAM E. ROBERTS, M.D.
Emeritus Professor of Otolaryngology,
University of Kansas Medical School,
Kansas City, Kansas

PREFACE

This book explains a new and, when fairly tried by physicians, highly successful method of treating and curing allergic diseases. As could be expected, some doctors have objected to any change in the conventional routine employed in the treatment of allergic patients for the past thirty or forty years.

During the last fifteen or twenty years I have talked with scores of physicians regarding the way allergic cases were being treated. I have found among doctors a general lack of enthusiasm about the procedures used in allergy cases. Many of them commented on the usual failures of physicians to give more than some partial, temporary relief to allergics.

Many brilliant and highly skilled physicians have difficulty in expressing medical terms, experiences, and opinions in language easily understandable by laymen. Most of their writings are for medical journals or medical books to be read by other doctors who would be bored by articles written for the general reading public.

What has been done in this book is to take available articles from medical journals dealing with the adrenal cortex extract or hypoadrenocorticism plan of treatment for allergic diseases, and rewrite them in language any intelligent layman can understand without having to resort to medical dictionaries and without having to ask for explanations from physicians.

I am deeply indebted to many wonderful doctors who, without charge, gladly helped me obtain medical material relating to hypoadrenocorticism (adrenal cortex insufficiency) and hypoglycemia (low blood sugar), and patiently answered my many questions regarding these subjects.

Even after I had written the book, I could never have published it had not a dozen or more of the nation's greatest physicians read copies of the first draft of the manuscript and given me suggestions and corrections which I incorporated into the text. To these dedicated doctors, not one of whom charged me a reading fee, I shall always be thankful.

Tom R. Blaine

GOODBYE ALLERGIES

1.

MORE MISERABLE THAN SICK

IF YOU ARE one of the nearly eighteen million known sufferers from allergic diseases in the United States, I bring you a message of hope and cheer. You can be cured of your allergies, or, if not cured, your health can be so much improved that your allergic diseases will cause you little or no concern.

Why am I so emphatic in saying you can be restored to such a marvelous state of health? After suffering from what the doctors called multiple allergies for more than sixty years, I was cured by a diet and medication given me by my family physician. Thousands of other allergy patients in all parts of the nation have been cured in the same manner.

This new treatment of allergies is one of the miracles of modern medicine. It is not a fad; it promotes nothing for sale; it was not thought up by medical charlatans; it does not require the services of a high-priced specialist; the drugs can be administered by your own physician as well as by any other doctor, and the diet can be followed easily.

From my allergists I learned that the word "allergy"

denotes a condition in which the response of an organism alters after contact with a foreign substance. An allergy, then, is an abnormal reaction of living tissues exposed to a specific substance. Yet the offending thing, the allergen, may produce no unfavorable reaction in a majority of people. It is not poisonous or pernicious *per se*.

The most common type of allergy is hay fever, known medically as allergic rhinitis. Seasonal hay fever is usually caused by hypersensitivity to the pollens of grasses, weeds, and trees at certain seasons of the year. Perennial hay fever may occur at any time or continue throughout the year. It may result from what we breathe, what we eat, drugs, chemicals, and from plants with which we come in contact. We are told we may be sensitive to changes in the weather, sunlight, gas fumes, and many other things. There seems to be no limit to the number of substances that may be harmful to us if we are sensitive to one or more of the known allergens. We may even be sensitive to cold—a physical allergy.

The sting of a bee or a wasp will make me ill. Once, while working in my back yard, I was stung by a wasp and my neighbor, a doctor working in his yard, hurriedly gave me an injection of an antihistamine which soon over-came the allergic reaction.

Fungus spores, the dander of animals (including house pets), feathers, dusts, flavoring and preservative materials, and serums are some of the more common allergens. Practically any food we eat or drink may act as an allergen. Milk, eggs, wheat, and white potatoes head the lists of foods which may cause allergic difficulties.

We have been taught that most, but by no means all, allergens are proteins. We have found from our experiences that we can suffer from asthma, migraine headache, hives, eczema, and many other allergic diseases, because of something we have eaten or inhaled, or because of something with which we have merely come in contact. I was told by a physician that I should avoid silk and woolen materials. I had just been informed by the same doctor that my skin tests revealed I was hypersensitive to so many different foods that I wondered if there were enough foods to which I was not allergic to keep me alive. To make my day perfect, I was told that I might later become hypersensitive to any food I was then permitted to eat!

Usually, allergies are diagnosed by means of a detailed history and skin tests. Intracutaneous injections and scratches are made to determine a negative or a positive reaction to all suspected foods, inhalants, and other substances. In my own case, skin tests revealed sensitivity to so many different things that the doctors admitted they were of little value. After years of these tests, I found that the only diagnostic method of any value to me as to foods, was an "off and on" experimentation with many different foods. However, allergy to foods may exist even when skin tests are negative!

After eliminating this and that food from my diet, later adding one and then another of the omitted foods, I found I could not tolerate any food generally known to cause allergies. In addition to those already named, I was not supposed to eat chocolate, several kinds of fruit, peanuts, tomatoes, and certain other foods.

My doctors informed me that if I would drop one of my allergic foods from my diet for a period of months I would become desensitized to it and it would probably cause me no further trouble when I started to eat it again. After years of attempting to desensitize against my enemy foods, the only change I noted, if any, was that I was more sensitive to them than before I had dropped them from my diet.

Doctors have said the histamine released by the sensitized cells, upon our exposure to allergens, causes us to have hay fever, asthma, migraine, skin eruptions, or whatever manifestation of allergies we may have. Most of us got tremendous temporary relief from our allergic symptoms by taking the antihistamines prescribed for us.

We have found that there is a hereditary predisposition toward allergies; that is, they run in families. We have also observed that when we have some emotional problems, when we are overworked or when things don't go as we expect, our allergies are worse. If we enjoyed a period of time in which there was little stress or strain, our allergic disorders usually improved. The emotional variable has been very confusing to those allergists who believe that contact of some part of our bodies with allergens is the cause of all allergic diseases. Some doctors have theorized that allergies are caused mentally and should be treated by removing the patient's deepseated emotional problems.

Many of the treatments employed during the past thirty-five years for people who are ill and sometimes barely able to stay up and around, seemed to me to have been rather primitive. For two years I took weekly injections of preparations supposedly made of the particular inhalants and contactants to which I was sensitive. These "shots," I was told, would desensitize me against the pollens, dusts, feathers, and animal dandruffs which caused me so much trouble. After twenty-four months of torture, with no beneficial results, I decided I had enough "desensitization."

About that time, I was given an adrenalin kit and told to give myself a hypodermic injection of adrenalin when breathing became difficult. I returned the kit after having tried to use it for three weeks, stating that I would just as soon be dead as to have to use that needle all of the time.

At another time, my nasal passages were cauterized with some sort of solution which made me feel that a red-hot rod had been thrust into each nostril. My rhinitis, or hay fever, was much worse after the cauterization.

It was suggested to me several times that my allergies probably were the result of unsolved emotional conflicts and that psychiatry might give me some relief. By that time I was so disgusted with the allergists' theories and beliefs that, fortunately for me, I did not waste any of my modest earnings on psychiatric treatments for my allergic diseases.

I know some allergy sufferers who have actually been given shock treatments. Many have undergone useless and unnecessary surgery which only aggravated their allergic conditions and made it more difficult than ever for them to achieve normal health.

My authority for the preceding statement is the April, 1963, issue of the *Reader's Digest*—a very conservative magazine—which carries, on page 151, a condensed article from the April *Family Doctor*, the official publication of the British Medical Association. On page 154 the writer states: "A famous survey revealed shocking facts: some 78 percent of ovaries removed were found to be perfectly normal; and some 30 percent of the uteri had nothing wrong with them. Most of this unnecessary surgery is performed in good faith. . . . One study followed 250 patients with gastrointestinal complaints but with no convincing evidence of organic disorder. More than half underwent operations which failed to relieve their symptoms. . . ."

You may have the impression this book was written for the purpose of attacking the medical profession. I hasten to assure you that such was not my intention. I was reared with the belief that two people are always right: my minister and my doctor. I sincerely believe that more than 95 per cent of all physicians and surgeons are high-class, conscientious, and dedicated men and women.

Twenty years' experience as a practicing attorney and nearly a quarter of a century on a state district court bench have given me some insight into what goes on in the minds of physicians. I have found they are just as human as the rest of us. This was forcibly brought home to me by a conversation I had some years ago with a physician. We had been talking about why doctors dislike to testify in court cases, and he asked if I knew the reason. I said I knew why lawyers believe doctors hate to be examined and cross-examined in court. "The lawyers are completely wrong," he replied. "No qualified physician has any serious fear of being 'shown up' before a court or a jury. He will be examined on a subject in which he is an expert. The lawyers know next to nothing about what the doctors have spent years learning. In his office or in the hospital the doctor makes the decisions and gives the orders. In a courtroom the doctor is pretty much like any other witness. There are others who make the decisions and give the orders, and doctors don't like to be placed in that kind of role. That is the reason why they hate to go to court."

The difficulty with the theories held by many allergists, that we can be desensitized against allergens, or that allergies are produced by mental or emotional disturbances, is this: *These theories sound wonderful, but they won't work.* Even if such theories had merit, it would be impossible in most cases to identify every food or foreign body to which we are sensitive; and no person, whether he suffers from allergies or not, can lead such a Spartan life that he never is subject to stress and strain, always has his emotions under control, and never allows any incident to disturb him. Even that effort would put him under stress!

A question the allergists have never answered to my satisfaction is this: "Why do only certain people have allergies?" I have read that skin tests show most individuals are sensitive to some foreign matter. Our bodies are invaded by outside substances to which skin tests show we are sensitive, yet, only a low percentage of people develop allergic diseases. It has always seemed to me that if we can find the answer to the above question, we will know the real cause of allergic diseases.

Before I was cured of allergies, I found I could get along fairly well by observing a lot of rules I had learned from a trial and error procedure. Oranges and grapefruit

never caused me trouble, but canned citrus fruit juice of
any kind gave me plenty of difficulty. On a business trip
to southern Texas, I asked a manufacturer of canned juices
if he knew why I could only tolerate fresh fruit or hand-
squeezed juices. He said it was impossible to manufacture
citrus fruit juices without getting some of the ground-up
seeds and peel in the processed products. He suggested
that I eat some orange seeds and peelings to see what, if
anything, would develop. I followed his suggestion and the
next day I had a severe rhinitis and an eczema over most
of my body.

Milk has always been one of my allergic foods, yet I always drank it since I felt I had to have its calcium and
phosphorus. I was most allergic to pasteurized milk, and
a little less sensitive to raw and canned milk. I found a
particular brand—dry, powdered, and nonfat—which I
seemed to be able to tolerate better than any other kind.
Since I had to take antihistamines even with this dry form,
I always drank my daily supply of milk at one time. I also
drank a prepared soybean milk, since it was supposed to
have many of the properties of cow's milk.

I learned that some foods would cause me little or no
trouble if taken alone, but would trigger some severe
allergic attacks in combinations of two or three. I had to
be careful to avoid sudden chills, although I have gotten
my voice back many times by breathing the fumes from
boiling water containing tincture of benzoin compound,
and then taking repeated icy showers.

I think it is generally conceded that there are two basic
types of food allergy: (1) *fixed* type, which is always

manifest when the particular food is ingested, and (2) *cyclical* type, in which the food—if sensitivity to it is mild —can be dropped from use for a long time and then reintroduced in the diet in small quantities and infrequently without giving rise to allergenic reaction. (There is only one trouble—it rarely works.)

The target organs of food allergy may be anywhere in the body: skin (eczema); respiratory system (asthma); gastrointestinal (diarrhea, etc.); genitourinary (urinary frequency and burning); and others.

Food control of allergies is not new. Coca demonstrated it in the 1920's, as did Rowe about 1931 in his publication, *Food Allergy.* During the past twenty-five years, so many doctors have recognized that allergies may be controlled by diet that this method of treatment now has the aura of tradition.

The plan of treatment later to be presented is a new modification of an accepted medical approach. An understanding of some fundamental medical truths regarding the functioning of the glands is a prerequisite to an explanation of how allergies can be eliminated by diet and medication.

Many allergy sufferers are sensitive to the chemical additives in foods rather than to the foods themselves. Since World War II, sodium propionates have been widely used as preservatives for cheese, bread, and tobacco. The propionates occur naturally in some forms of cheese, such as Swiss cheese. For those who cannot tolerate the propionates, the result is an intestinal allergy in which migraine is common.

If, after having eaten a good dinner in the evening, one should develop an allergic attack after midnight or near morning, he should determine if propionates are causing the attacks. I know a man who frequently, after eating a steak dinner, had a severe migraine about three o'clock the next morning. He recalled that at each dinner preceding the migraine he had used a blue cheese salad dressing. When he discontinued eating cheese, he had no more migraine.

Another friend complained about the onset of hay fever some mornings at five o'clock. She had never before suffered from allergies and remembered that her only change in eating habits was that she had started eating cheese before retiring. When she stopped eating cheese the hay fever disappeared.

As a young man, I often had sores in my mouth and nothing the doctors prescribed helped to heal them. A few years ago I discovered that the sores were caused by an allergy to aspirin.

Because of my sensitivity to gas fumes, we were never able to live in a home with open gas flames or with an ordinary gas floor furnace.

When I tried to discuss some of these things with physicians, I was usually met with a stock statement that many people have idiosyncrasies, and the best thing I could do was to get my mind off myself and lead as normal a life as possible. When a doctor got around to mentioning my "neurosis" or my "hypochondriac state," I was always ready to look for another doctor.

A diagnostician told me in 1931 that I was suffering from multiple allergies and sent me to an allergy clinic.

The early thirties were memorable years for more than the great depression which made earning a living difficult for nearly all of us. It was a time when unadulterated Freudianism was popular with both doctors and laymen. Only about half of the medical schools in America then offered regular courses in psychosomatic medicine; yet doctors who had never taken the equivalent of an advanced course in psychology were diagnosing their allergic patients as suffering from psychoneurosis, and sending them to psychiatrists for treatment.

In 1935, I went to Oklahoma City to see a noted surgeon whom I had known for years, since he came from my home town. I knew he suffered from as many allergies as I did, so my visit to him was primarily to get sympathy. My friend, Dr. Patrick Nagle, said to me:

"You have been to the allergy clinics in Oklahoma and to the big-name clinics out of the state and you are right back where you started.

"Don't make the mistake of running from doctor to doctor, trying to get relief from your allergies. All we can do is to try to help you on a day-to-day basis. You are less of a neurotic than any other allergy patient I have, so you can forget about neurosis. When a doctor tells a patient he is suffering from a neurosis, you can often be sure the doctor is just trying to cover up his own ignorance.

"Be your own doctor. All we doctors know now about allergies is how to help our patients avoid the causes of their illnesses. I admit it is a crude method of treatment, but until medical science comes up with something better, we will have to continue in this manner.

"My opinion, for whatever it is worth, is that we are

treating the symptoms instead of the causes of allergies. You and I will see the day, in all probability, when allergies will be cured. I think it will come through the work of biochemists and endocrinologists.

"I recommend that you make a study of nutrition. We doctors know little or nothing about nutrition; yet it is very important in allergy cases."

Dr. Nagle died of cancer before any cure for allergic diseases had been perfected; his words were prophetic. From the day I talked with him, I was convinced that medical science would eventually cure my allergic diseases.

I always had the impression that some time my local doctor would call me and say: "Tom, a successful means of curing allergies is now available. When do you want to start your treatments?" The cure was not that prosaic, but came rather dramatically as you will later learn. Not only did I get over my allergic diseases, but I gained dynamic and vigorous health at a time when I was near the Biblical three score and ten years.

It seems to me this would be a good time to take a look at ourselves and see what kind of people we, who are subject to allergies, are. We have been told by our doctors that we have relatively higher intelligence than most people. We are usually rather meticulous in our work—perfectionists who sometimes drive ourselves to exhaustion. Our doctors frequently complain that we do not know the meaning of the word relaxation.

In addition to suffering from our specific allergies, we often are nervous, irritable, and apprehensive, and complain to our doctors of weakness, fatigue, depression, and insomnia, especially after physical, emotional or infectious stress. We are frequently treated for low blood pressure and anemia, usually bruise easily because of capillary fragility, and frequently seem to be either too hot or too cold when others appear to be comfortable. We think we have a fever, only to find that our body temperature is one or two degrees below normal.

Often, the women among us tend to be flat chested, whereas the men frequently have little hair on their chests or on the lateral two-thirds of their legs. We usually have an abundant head of fine hair and, when we arise after a night's rest, a puffiness under our eyes.

There are spells in which our appetites drive us to eat exorbitant amounts of foods, especially carbohydrates; at times we have a terrific craving for sugar or salt. Experience has taught us that our allergies are worse when we eat an excessive amount of carbohydrates, yet we seem to be powerless to resist huge amounts of starches and sugars, or products made from starch or sugar.

Well aware that we should exercise daily, we feel too tired from what we must do to exert ourselves unnecessarily. The typical allergic or hypoadrenocortic patient is lean, although some have weight problems they cannot solve. We are constantly reminded that we should eat less and we know we are overweight; yet we don't get enough energy from the foods we eat—excessive in amount as they may be—to do the things we have to, much less the many other things we would like to do.

Our doctors experiment on us and give us the usual medications for infectious diseases without any resulting

benefits. Although we pay doctors better than do the
average nonallergic patients, we frequently have the feeling that we are not too welcome in our doctors' offices.
What allergy sufferer hasn't at some time heard a receptionist say on the telephone or interoffice communication
system: "That Mrs. Brown with her awful headache is
here. How do you want me to get rid of her, doctor?"

Most of us believed the miracle drugs of this era would
cure our allergies, but in that we were disappointed. We
watched, with interest and enthusiasm, the progress medicine was making on all fronts in curing the infectious
diseases and felt we were the stepchildren of medicine.
Sometimes we have been tempted to believe that we are
the forgotten people of medicine.

Some of the wealthier victims of seasonal allergies are
able to go to different regions to escape the suffering of
those who cannot afford to change their climate; air con-
ditioning helps many others during the pollen seasons. We
benefit by taking vitamin food supplements, but we sometimes find we are sensitive to some of the pharmaceutical
preparations out of which vitamins are made.

Dieting has always been boring to me although I have
had a weight problem since I was thirty years old. Actually, I never "dieted" until I started the diet which, with
the prescribed medication, got me over my allergies and
gave me real health. Before that, I alternately starved or
gorged. The diet I will tell you about is the only one I
ever heard of for obese persons that is worth the paper it
is written on. If you are inclined to be overweight, this
diet will be like something sent from Heaven. You can

eat three meals a day, have snacks between meals and at bedtime, and not gain weight. That hungry feeling you have had while trying to lose weight will soon be gone, probably forever.

I am certain you will be as enthusiastic about the treatments as I was, and for the first time in your life, you will have the grand and glorious feeling that comes when you realize your allergies are disappearing. You will keep saying to yourself, as I did: "Can this wonderful feeling of well-being be real?" When a friend remarks to you, "I never saw you looking better," you will be glad you are alive and thankful to those pioneers in medical science who made your relief from allergic suffering possible.

2.

YOUR AMAZING GLANDS

YOUR ENDOCRINE SYSTEM of glands consists of the adrenal glands, the pituitary gland, the thyroid gland, the pancreas gland with its islands of Langerhans, the pineal gland and the sex glands. These glands are also referred to as the endocrine or ductless glands because, unlike exocrine or sweat glands, they send their secretions inside the body.

The pituitary gland is a pea-sized powerhouse attached to the brain stem; one of its important functions is to regulate and secrete our growth hormones. The thyroid gland—resembling a small oyster in shape—is located deep in the throat; it provides chemicals which control metabolism and help us deal with emotional stress. Embedded in the thyroid are the parathyroids, which remind us of BB shots. Most people have four parathyroids, but some have only one and others have as many as eight.

The adrenals, each one above a kidney, look something like mushrooms. Actually, each adrenal consists of two glands, a cove (the medulla) and a casing (the cortex), like a nut and its husk. The adrenals are, in a sense, the "kings of the glands," as we shall soon see.

Little is known about the pineal gland except that it lies in the middle of the brain and has some influence on the functioning of the adrenals. The pancreas is six or eight inches long and resembles a bunch of grapes. Its primary function is to secrete fluids (hormones) which help us digest food. This gland is regulated by and owes its functional tone and vitality to the amazing chemical power of the adrenals, which influence many hormones.

Nearly a hundred years ago, a young medical student named Langerhans discovered a group of cells in the pancreas neither connected with nor related to the rest of the gland. Later it was discovered that these cells, or the islands of Langerhans (sometimes called the islets of the pancreas), produce the body's insulin. As described in our next chapter, insulin plays an important part in the successful treatment and cure of allergic diseases.

No one seems to know how many chemicals are secreted by any one endocrine gland. Doctors tell us they have found that the adrenals secrete at least thirty-two chemicals (hormones), and the pituitary gland secretes at least a dozen. Each of the other endocrines gives off at least one hormone, probably more.

The pituitary is constantly manufacturing and sending out chemicals to stir up the other endocrines, each of which reacts in the same manner. The command and response signals coordinate, speed up, or slow down our bodily and mental functions; they control digestion, the blood stream, the heart, and all of our thinking, feeling, and perceiving.

One pituitary hormone regulates the growth of an infant into an adult. If there is too little of this hormone, the child is a dwarf; if there is too much, the child becomes a giant. Formerly, when a baby was born with a nonfunctioning thyroid, he was doomed to be an idiot; but now, thanks to the endocrinologists, if a baby is born without a thyroid gland and is supplied regularly with the thyroid hormones of meat animals, he will develop into a normal adult.

The hormones of the adrenal cortex (the casing) are the most marvelous of all. They maintain life; without them we could not live, for they are the prime regulators of the chemical processes which convert what we eat and drink from chemical substances into useful materials for the functioning, repairing and rebuilding of our bodies.

If it were not for these adrenal cortex hormones, the proteins, fats, carbohydrates, and minerals which we ingest could never be converted into energy and body tissues. We know now that the involuntary (autonomic) nervous system and the endocrine system work together most intimately.

Suppose the body is under stress. The nerves send a message to the adrenal cores, which then secrete a chemical, adrenalin, into the bloodstream. This chemical steps up heart action and narrows the blood vessels so that the blood can be pushed through them with more force; simultaneously it relaxes and opens the air passageways to the

lungs so that more air can reach the lungs quickly. Adrenalin also stimulates the pituitary to send out hormones which cause the adrenal cortex and thyroid to secrete chemicals. Instantly this process prepares both body and mind to deal with the stress. It accounts for somewhat superhuman feats of strength and quick thinking and acting in an emergency.

You are already saying to yourself: "All of this is interesting reading and something we should know about our bodies, but what does it have to do with my allergies?" The answer is, it has much to do, not only with your allergies, but with your general health. Soon we will see how weak and damaged adrenals are responsible for your tired, worn-out, irritable, and depressed feelings.

I will explain why your efficiency is so low and your tendency to go to pieces is so great, and how your seeming inability to ever get things done is the result of an unhealthy endocrine system. You will be told how your personality can zoom, how you can regain a feeling of well-being and a zest for living and doing things—all by building up the adrenal glands.

Doctors tell us we are as old as our arteries, but I say we are as well as are our endocrines. It is my belief, based on my experience, that the greatest medical discovery of this age, as far as allergy sufferers are concerned, is that weak and diseased adrenal glands (even if inherited) can be made into healthy adrenals by medication and by a diet which does not place too much strain on them. *That, in a nutshell, is the story of this book.* The same things that are causing you to be weak, nervous, depressed, ap-

prehensive, and irritable are causing you to suffer from allergic diseases.

The endocrinologists set out to find ways and means to improve our general health by treating the endocrine system. In so doing (perhaps accidentally—I admit I don't know) they came up with the causes and cures for our allergic diseases.

The credit for the relief of allergic diseases rightfully belongs to those physicians and surgeons who work on the one big remaining frontier of medical science, endocrinology. The endocrinologists, like all great men of science, are very modest. They admit that what is not yet known about endocrinology may be more important than what is known. Still, they have pointed the way to health and strength for millions of us who have despaired of ever living normal and healthy lives.

We must remember that medical science has only lately become aware of the subtle workings and importance of the endocrines. This is not difficult to understand. These glands are in widely separated parts of the body; their appearances are not the same, and their secretions are heavily cloaked by chemical subtleties.

All of the body's other glands have ducts which carry their secretions to the places where they serve purposes; but nature has so well hidden the connections among the endocrines and their cooperative efforts that it is a medical marvel that the endocrinologists have discovered so much of her secrets.

In the succeeding chapters, I will attempt to show you, how these wonderful endocrine glands make and keep us

the persons we are, well or ill, and how they determine whether we are pleasant or unpleasant, calm or jittery, energetic or always tired. But most important of all, you will see how simple and easy it is to get and maintain a healthy endocrine system, and how, when this is accomplished, your allergies will disappear!

When, in 1959, my local doctor handed me a medical journal and for the first time in my life I read that *allergies were being cured,* I was so excited I could not leave the chair in the doctor's office until I had read the entire article. It was certainly something different from what I had been told in the thirties and forties, such as: "Your allergies are something you are going to have to live with the rest of your life. . . . If you are careful of what you eat and if you avoid the pollens and dusts to which you are sensitive, you should live to a reasonable old age. . . . There is sometimes a tendency to outgrow some allergies. We hope that will be true in your case. . . . I think you spend too much time thinking and talking about your allergies. Maybe more outside activities will help you."

I have no bitterness toward any doctor who treated me for allergies. I got the finest he was able to give and his charges were always reasonable. Without the help of these physicians, I would never have been able to continue in my chosen profession. Certainly, none of them can be criticized for not attempting to find a cure for allergies before the means for effecting the cure were known.

In 1933 one doctor advised me that there was a definite connection between calcium deficiency and my perennial hay fever. He prescribed calcium gluconate wafers, which

I took for more than a year until an allergy specialist in Chicago informed me that calcium gluconate was worthless and recommended I discontinue taking it.

Now we are told that low blood sugar is usually accompanied by low serum calcium and that introducing calcium into an antihypoglycemia diet or injecting it into the patient's system hastens recovery from the deficiency. This is always recommended, so I have read, where the tests show low calcium serum.

Also valuable were the warnings the doctors gave me shortly before I went on the diet and took the medication which cured my allergies. I was desperate for any kind of help I could get, since my general health had so deteriorated that I was not certain I would be able to continue my work as district judge in a large district. New oil fields were being discovered in all of the counties I served. Litigation was increasing everywhere in my judicial district. I dragged myself home after a day's work with only one thought, getting enough rest so I could try to do the next day's work. Since cortisone made me feel well, I begged several physicians to permit me to take it, but all of them warned me that the hormone could and would do me great harm.

One doctor said the use of cortisone was so dangerous that were I to take any appreciable amount I would have to carry a card stating that I was on cortisone. If I were to be injured in an automobile accident and given medication by someone who did not know I had recently taken cortisone, I might die.

Another physician warned me that if I took much cor-

tisone I might get what he called a "buffalo hump" on the back of my neck and my face could become deformed. I was also told cortisone might cause me to have a coronary thrombosis or, for that matter, thrombosis (blood clot) in any of my blood vessels. There were so many other warnings about serious dangers resulting from the use of cortisone that I completely gave up any thought of taking it.

If the adrenals are functioning normally they need no stimulation to make them secrete cortisone and other hormones. I understand, from what doctors have told me and from what I have read, that the adrenocorticotrophic hormone, ACTH, stimulates the adrenal glands—that it activates tired or nearly exhausted adrenals to produce a little more cortisone. However, the effect of ACTH on weakened adrenal glands—even when administered for a relatively short time—can be very harmful. In large doses, the hormone may produce adverse side effects (hypertension, muscle weakness, moonface, or acne) representing exaggerated physiological response.

Some means other than administering ACTH or cortisone must be employed to permit the adrenals to rehabilitate. They must be given a chance to rest and rebuild.

In the two following chapters I shall attempt to explain as best I can how some endocrinologists have discovered and worked out a program of diet and medication that allows nearly exhausted adrenals to regain more tone without ceasing their activities (which would result from large doses of cortisone). I hope this will prove as fascinating to you as it was to me when I was researching all available publications and interviewing as many doctors as would allow me to ask them questions.

Many sins have been committed unintentionally against persons who had one or more endocrine disorders. As we will later see, these people were not informed by their doctors of the cause of their depressed and sometimes despondent feelings.

Since I have been a judge, I have heard more divorce cases than all other civil and criminal cases combined; more than 50 per cent of all cases filed in my courts have been divorce cases. Here is the testimony in a typical divorce case brought before me by a wife: The husband complains of being tired and worn out, is unable to get and keep a job, and has some allergic disorders, but his doctors have been unable to find anything organically wrong with him that should prevent him from being regularly employed. The wife's conclusions are that her husband is lazy, worthless, and a liability instead of an asset. She tells the court that it is enough for her to have to support herself and her two children, and that if she can win a divorce there will be one less mouth to feed.

When the husband institutes the divorce case against his wife, his proof runs something like this: The wife has become a sloppy and indifferent housekeeper who con-constantly complains of exhaustion. She spends too much time, so her husband says, in bed and doesn't even take good care of her own personal appearance, much less the children. She apparently has lost her interest in living and readily admits that all charges made against her are true —that the doctors found nothing organically wrong with her, that the medicines she took for her headaches and sinus attacks didn't do any good. She realizes she spends too much money for vitamin pills and overeats. She confesses she doesn't know what is the matter with her.

You are ready to say to me: "You are a judge, not a doctor. How can you know what is wrong with these unhappy and seemingly worthless people who go through your divorce courts?" That is a fair question, and I will try to answer it. I insisted on having many of these people take glucose tolerance tests and a complete blood count. When my suggestion was followed and it was found that the husband or wife needed medication and a diet for an endocrine gland condition, it was not long before we had a different husband or wife; a home which had been ready to fall apart at the seams was saved.

In one case the wife was fat, unattractive, and indifferent about her home at the time of divorce. After following a proper diet and taking medication prescribed by a doctor who wasn't blindly prejudiced against a treatment he had never used before, she made a phenomenal recovery in a short time and she and her husband came back to court to have the divorce decree vacated.

As I shall later explain, my studies have convinced me that many of the drinking problems of the husbands, wives, and parents who come to the divorce courts are related to endocrine diseases, either inherited or acquired. Our endocrine glands can make or break us.

Since this is a book dealing largely with the endocrines, I assure you I did not submit the manuscript for publication until several reputable physicians had read it and had given me the benefit of their suggestions. The opinions I give about physicians are my own, but any statement in the book regarding diet, disease, diagnosis, medication, or any other phase of medical practice, has the approval of these physicians and may be accepted by you as if it had been written by a medical specialist in the subject under discussion.

3.

HYPOGLYCEMIA, A NEW NAME
FOR AN OLD DISEASE

HYPOGLYCEMIA IS A low blood sugar condition, the opposite of hyperglycemia, a condition in which there is excess sugar in the bloodstream.

Hyperinsulinism is a medical term used to describe a condition caused by an excessive secretion of insulin by those parts of the pancreas called the islands of Langerhans. Unfortunately, some members of the medical profession will not accept the term "hyperinsulinism" and prefer to call the condition "relative hypoglycemia." It was interesting to note that in some recent medical articles the terms "functional hyperinsulinism" and "relative hypoglycemia" were used interchangeably. Hyperinsulinism results in a low blood sugar—hypoglycemia. It is the opposite of diabetes—high blood sugar resulting from an insufficient secretion of the hormone insulin.

When the islands of Langerhans cannot produce enough insulin the result is diabetes—too much sugar in the bloodstream. The conversion of foods, especially carbohydrates, into blood sugar or glucose keeps the sugar level high. The principle behind urine tests for diabetes is that when the blood sugar rises high enough, some of it spills into the urine.

Hyperinsulinism (too much insulin—the opposite of diabetes) has been called the hunger disease, the starvation disease, and the fatigue disease. An abnormal hunger, sometimes of a most ravenous kind, particularly for sugar, is often characteristic of a low blood sugar condition. Chronic fatigue is the commonest complaint.

In their book, *Body, Mind and Sugar,* Abrahamson and Pezet say: "Perhaps, hyperinsulinism will in time be known as sugar starvation, for that is what it literally is. Sugar is the fuel of every cell in the body. While most body cells can derive some nourishment from other sources, however, the nourishment of the brain is exclusively glucose."

The last statement explains why we who have low blood sugar, or hyperinsulinism, or hypoglycemia, have so many headaches. Our brains, as well as our bodies, are crying out for nourishment—glucose.

Because diabetes, if not controlled, may result in death, much attention has been paid to high blood sugar by the medical profession for many years. Some doctors estimate there may be three to six times as many sufferers from low blood sugar as there are known diabetics, and yet, low blood sugar continues to be largely ignored by the men and women of medical science. Let me explain what I mean by a striking example: *Gray's Attorney's Textbook of Medicine,* a very fine work consisting of three large volumes, is in every law library and perhaps half of the offices of practicing attorneys in all the states.

In the index of *Gray's Attorney's Textbook of Medicine* we find that the entry for diabetes consists of 85 lines and takes up almost a page. Low blood sugar is disposed of in the text (Sec. 133.15, page 1402) in exactly seventeen words, as follows: "Hypoglycemia is a decreased amount of sugar in the blood. These people are usually irascible, undesirable employees."

When I inquired of physicians about the reason low blood sugar sufferers have, for the most part, been tossed into the medical waste baskets, I received no satisfactory answers. Dr. Sidney A. Portis of the medical faculty of the University of Illinois believes the difficulty is that the cure for low blood sugar "cannot be packaged, publicized, and sold over the counter in a drug store." Dr. E. M. Abrahamson, a noted diabetes specialist, thought that if low blood sugar could be cured by a miracle drug, or if there were some glamorous manner in which physicians could package and prescribe a cure, the doctors would show more enthusiasm in trying to do something for low blood sugar sufferers. Another doctor I recently spoke with said, "Frankly, I don't think a lot of doctors know how to diagnose and treat hypoglycemia."

It is difficult for a layman to understand why many doctors seem to have a prejudice against hypoglycemia. If physicians will only think of hypoglycemia as they do of other bodily ailments, they might be able to diagnose it more readily and learn how to treat it more effectively.

Although many excellent articles have appeared in recent

years in the medical journals, explaining why hypoglycemia sufferers cannot eat quickly absorbed carbohydrate foods, *some doctors still prescribe sugar for hypoglycemia, which is the worst thing they can do since sugar primes the pancreas to secrete more insulin, thus actually making the hypoglycemia worse.* Only the well-informed doctor will treat hypoglycemia with a low carbohydrate, high protein diet. He knows that unless patients are willing to change their self-indulgent habits during the time they are being cured, they will continue to complain of hunger, fatigue, anxiety, and nervousness, perhaps along with crying spells, headaches, mental confusion, and all kinds of allergic disorders.

It is easier to prescribe antihistamines or some tranquilizing medicine than it is to go through the long ordeal of persuading patients to meet the facts squarely—to give up what they have always been taught were innocent and harmless foods which they prize highly. With many patients, it will be a long selling job on the part of the doctor to even get them in a frame of mind to try to trade some of their supposedly innocent eating and drinking habits for good health.

Let us have a look at the kind of people who are "usually irascible, undesirable employees." Low blood sugar sufferers are found in all of the professions, including medicine. They usually have superior intelligence and better than average education. They are the thinkers and the doers of our country. Among the laboring people, low blood sugar sufferers are the ones who are highly skilled. You see them in large numbers among the "white collar" workers, the writers, the artists, the people in show business, in fact, in all walks of life. Even when not cured, these people frequently live to advanced years because they generally take good care of their health as far as they know how. Also, as physicians have told me, their tissues age more slowly than do the tissues of other persons because of their particular body metabolism.

Most low blood sugar patients are ambitious and inherently aggressive, and although they are more introverted than extroverted, they usually like other people. Possibly their strangest characteristic is their refusal to recognize defeat when the odds all seem to be against them. They carry on their chosen occupations and support themselves and their families long after those with normal blood sugar have given up. Their "do or die" determination, once they have made up their minds to do something, is a valuable asset to the physician in helping them to be restored to good health.

We have talked in general terms of the principal complaints of the hypoglycemics. These are by no means all of the symptoms of low blood sugar disease. Doctors have told me these people sometimes feel lightheaded and exhausted. They occasionally lose consciousness if the glucose starvation of the brain is severe. Some of them may have had brain surgery when there was nothing wrong with the brain. Doctors report palpitation of the heart followed by convulsions. While I was suffering from hyperinsulinism I had several insulin shocks. However, I did not know until I had been cured of low blood sugar and had read every article I could find on the subject that the frightening experiences I had were insulin shocks. My doctors thought I might have had some slight strokes. I was afraid they were heart attacks, even though all tests showed otherwise.

There is another blood sugar condition known as dysinsulinism in which the tests may show the patient has alternately low and then high blood sugar. Some members of the medical profession who do not accept the term "hyperinsulinism" and prefer to say "relative hypoglycemia" instead, may challenge the use of the word "dysinsulinism" in describing a condition alternating between low and high blood sugar. I cannot see how it makes much difference what the doctors call these abnormal conditions as long as they are properly diagnosed and correctly treated.

I was introduced to hyperinsulinism in 1950, when I had been assigned to hold court for a week in one of the larger cities of our state. We completed the trial of a jury case on Monday and the next morning I had one of the worst migraine headaches I have ever experienced. The right side of my head had that throbbing sensation (more like a pounding feeling) with which I was so familiar, and I felt sick all over. A local district judge offered to take over my bench since his cases for the day had been settled, and he recommended that I take the day off after seeing his family doctor. I went to my hotel room and tried to sleep, but the migraine pains were too severe for me to stay in bed. I called the judge's doctor and he told me to come out to his office and that he would see me right away.

The doctor's receptionist led me into his office a few minutes after I arrived. I expected him to give me the usual sedative, a prescription for antihistamines, and a short lecture on not being so tense. His examination was brief—a few questions about what I ate on Monday and where the pains were in my head. "I think we can get you over this migraine attack before evening, maybe sooner," he remarked casually. "Your blood sugar level is too low. When we get it back where it should be, you will feel fine. I am going to have my nurse give you three antihistamine tablets and three aspirins. I want you to take two of each of them now and in about an hour or so take the other two. As soon as you can, I want you to drink two or three cups of black coffee with no sugar. Then go to a grocery store, get some unsweetened fruit; dried apricots or dried peaches will do. After you have eaten the fruit, you should take a brisk walk for thirty to forty-five minutes. When you have taken the last aspirin and antihistamine tablet, go to your room and to bed. If you can sleep a couple of hours, you should feel fine."

He asked me if I knew anything about low blood sugar and I confessed that I knew nothing about it. He said that his wife had migraine and he had found the plan recommended to me beneficial to her. "What has happened," he said, "is that you have eaten too much carbohydrate, especially sugar. A part of your pancreatic gland is too sensitive; when you eat starch or sugar or both, too much insulin is produced in response to your body's demand and it literally eats up your blood sugar, or glucose. This is why migraine sufferers are nearly always hungry. Your blood

sugar is deficient and you feel terrible. It is the sudden-
ness of the fall of the blood sugar which brings on migraine. Everything I have told you to do should raise the
level of your blood sugar. The fruit you eat will be
absorbed slowly, not fast enough to bring about a lot more
insulin secretion."

"Doctor," I asked, "you mean this terrible headache
wasn't caused by some stress or strain, as I have been told
by doctors all these years?" "Oh, stress and strain do have
some effect on the pancreas and cause more insulin to be
secreted," he answered. "But I don't think migraine can
always be classed as an emotional ailment. I can see how
easy it would be for one suffering from migraine to become emotional."

I mentioned to him that I usually had a premonition
that I was going to have a migraine attack. "This premonition you talk about is caused by the chemical changes
taking place in your body. You remember how you felt
before you had an attack in the past. Somewhere along
the line, before your brain gives that distress signal that
it isn't getting enough glucose, you know from past experiences you are going to have migraine. My patients
don't all experience for the same length of time the warnings that all is not well with the blood sugar."

After drinking the coffee, taking the medicine, eating
the fruit, and finishing the walk, I went to my hotel room.
In a few minutes I was sleeping and did not wake up for
nearly three hours. When I got up, I felt wonderful but
hungry. I celebrated my first real victory over migraine
by going out and eating the biggest steak I could find.

After that, when I knew a migraine attack was coming, I followed the same routine the doctor had recommended and always got over the headaches before they wore me out. Before I learned about low blood sugar, a migraine headache sometimes lasted two or three days.

Since coffee is not on the hypoglycemic's diet, you may wonder why it was prescribed for migraine, which is a severe hypoglycemic attack. The pain of a migraine is so severe, and the suffering so great, that ordinary pain killers are wholly ineffective; the sufferer cannot wait several hours for blood sugar to gradually find its way into his bloodstream. Caffeine causes elevation of the blood sugar level soon after it is taken, and also stimulates the adrenal glands to release adrenalin, which helps smother the excessive insulin in the bloodstream.

Under normal circumstances, a hypogylcemic does not drink coffee because he does not want the supply of glycogen stored in his liver (and available as glucose or blood sugar in an emergency) dissipated by caffeine. Neither does he desire to stimulate his adrenal glands to produce more adrenalin.

Any person who has ever experienced a severe migraine will agree that it is not a normal circumstance and that emergency measures for relief are always justified. The migraine sufferer needs blood sugar and adrenalin released into his bloodstream as quickly as it can be done.

One patient told me that when he felt an attack coming on, he drank several cups of strong black coffee and ate two or three pieces of hard sugar candy. I inquired if the candy caused him any bad aftereffects. "Yes," he said, "I am certain it causes me to feel more knocked out the next day, but it helps me get over the migraine quicker." I tried taking some sugar candy once with a severe migraine and I thought the sugar made the pain worse and the attack harder to overcome.

What we have been discussing is hypoglycemia which readily responds to a high protein, medium fat, low carbohydrate diet, and the medication recommended in the next chapter. The tests for hypoglycemia are the same as those for hypoadrenocorticism. If it is determined that a patient is not suffering from hypoglycemia but has hyperinsulinism resulting from a tumor or a growth on the islands of Langerhans, surgery is the only effective way to a cure.

I will say without equivocation that there have been more mistakes made in diagnosing the ailments of the people I have known who had low blood sugar than in diagnosing the ailments of any other similar number of ill people I ever heard of. They have been operated on and treated for about every disease on record. Since all such treatments are ineffective for a low blood sugar condition, there has always remained the "hysteria" or the "neurosis" diagnosis to fall back on.

These wretched, unfortunate, badly treated, but worthwhile men and women deserve more consideration from our well-intentioned doctors than they have been getting. These people, with their higher intelligence, their superior abilities, their determination to succeed when others would have given up, their high ideals, their loyalties to their families, and their willingness to conform to the requirements of our society, cannot be cast aside medically as if they were an unimportant segment of our population. They constitute the backbone of this country. It is as imperative that they be cured as it is that diabetics be permitted to live long, useful, and healthy lives.

The diet for low blood sugar must be one that will depress the already oversensitive islands of Langerhans. As we shall later see, it must be one that places as little strain as possible on the endocrines, particularly the adrenals. It must be high in protein but low in carbohydrates, and it must contain only those carbohydrates that are slowly absorbed. Remember, we are trying not to arouse the insulin-making islets of the pancreas. We must "slip up on" these islets of the pancreas with our carbohydrates.

Fats do not increase the activity of the insulin-making parts of our bodies, but we must be reasonable in our intake since excessive fats cause obesity, arteriosclerosis, and diabetes, as our doctors tell us. We certainly do not want to bring on any more ailments than we already have. Since we are trying to cure cell starvation, even when we are overweight, it is better that we eat frequently rather than depend on the conventional three meals daily.

On arising in the morning after a long fast, someone with low blood sugar will not have much pep or enthusiasm for the day's work. Coffee stimulates the adrenal cortex to produce more hormones and these hormones cause the liver to convert its glycogen into glucose; so, we get a lift from an early cup of coffee. The lift is of short duration, for the islets of the pancreas produce more than enough insulin to eat up, as it were, the glucose set free by the caffeine in the coffee; we need another cup of coffee while the liver's supply of stored glycogen is being dissipated by the in-sulin. Sugar gives us the same stimulating effect; but the glucose coming from the sugar meets the same fate as does the glucose coming from the liver's stored glycogen. What is even worse, the blood sugar (glucose) which was in the bloodstream before we ate the sugar or drank the coffee is used up by the insulin, and our blood sugar drops lower than it was before we drank the coffee or ate the sugar.

As you have already found from your experiences, and as appears logical from what has been said, someone with hyperinsulinism usually feels best after eating a good dinner in the evening.

Here is the diet I was on while being cured of my allergic diseases:

ANTIHYPOGLYCEMIA DIET

Foods Allowed:

All meats, fish, and shell fish.

Dairy products—eggs, milk, butter, and cheese.

Also recommended—1 pint to 1 quart of acidophilus milk daily.

Milk between meals; milk, cheese and/or butter and saltines before retiring.

All vegetables and fruits not listed below.

Salted nuts (excellent between meals).

Peanut butter.

Protein bread.

Soybeans and soybean products.

Decaffeinated coffee, weak tea, and sugar-free sodas

Saccharin or sodium cyclamate as a substitute for sugar.

(If one is on a salt controlled diet, he should use saccharin or calcium cyclamate.)

Foods to Avoid:

Potatoes, corn, macaroni, spaghetti, rice.

Pie, cake, pastries, sugar, candies.

Dates and raisins.

Cola and other sweet soft drinks.

Alcohol in all forms.

Coffee and strong tea.

All hot and cold cereals (except occasionally oat meal).

Having milk or fruits between meals is advisable in order to prevent blood sugar levels from slackening off (as is prone to occur two or three hours after meals). Ordinarily there is no restriction on salt intake; in fact, many doctors advise low blood sugar patients to take supplementary salt tablets, especially during hot weather, to replace the loss caused by perspiration.

The importance of adhering to this diet strictly cannot be overemphasized. Dietary indiscretions will cause a return of the hateful symptoms of a low blood sugar condition and the accompanying allergic disorders. Unless one has made up his mind to be cured of hypoglycemia and to stick with this diet at all times until the allergies are gone for good, he will be wasting the time of his doctor and his own time in starting the diet.

Probably the greatest difficulty is giving up coffee, but this is imperative. No intoxicating beverage of any kind in any amount may be taken. We must never forget that one of the reasons for following the diet and abstaining from alcohol or other intoxicants is to maintain the blood sugar at a proper level. What we must achieve is an appropriate balance between the sugar-repressing actions of the islands of Langerhans and the sugar-releasing functions of the hormones from the adrenal cortex. We should also remember that some of the hormones secreted by the adrenals actually smother the excessive insulin of the islets of the pancreas when we suffer from hyperinsulinism.

I appreciate the fact that diagnosis of hypoglycemia is not a cut and dried process with physicians. I also understand that many doctors, otherwise well qualified, have not had extensive training in endocrinologic precepts. The symptoms and complaints of the patients are generally vague and indefinite. A patient will tell his physician he is suffering from sinus trouble, severe headaches, or abdominal pains. The doctor knows the patient came to him for treatment for his sinus difficulty, his headaches or his abdominal pains, and too frequently the doctor tries to treat the particular part of the body about which complaint is made. As a layman who has experienced most of the problems of health discussed in this book and was finally restored to robust health, I think the greatest weakness of modern day physicians is their tendency to consider any illness which is difficult to diagnose properly as emotional in character and then attempt to treat the patient accordingly.

I tried to get relief from my migraine headaches from at least ten doctors, and all of them talked about my reaction to stress. They were right in one sense; my reaction to stress was poor because of inadequate hormone production by my adrenals and an excessive hormone production (of insulin) by the islets of my pancreas. I accidentally went to a physician who knew why my reaction to stress was not good because of special studies he had made to assist his wife in getting over migraine attacks.

Physicians, however, have this advantage: even a perfunctory questioning of hypoglycemics will disclose they all have a myriad of common complaints, such as fatigue, weakness, depression, insomnia, nervousness, and apprehensiveness. They will all say these symptoms are much worse following physical, emotional, or infectious stress.

4.

HYPOADRENOCORTICISM—
YOU MAY HAVE IT

DR. JOHN W. TINTERA, an outstanding endocrinol-
ogist, has defined hypoadrenocorticism as encountered in
allergy cases as "subclinical Addison's disease." Addison's
disease is a disease of the adrenal cortex characterized by
extremely low blood sugar. It is not common, fortunately,
but until comparatively recent years was considered incurable. Persons suffering from this disease acquire a dark
pigmentation of the skin, suffer from low blood pressure,
have weak muscles, and frequently are emaciated. The
word "subclinical" usually denotes a period prior to the
appearance of manifest symptoms in the evolution of a
disease.

Recently I read a very old medical book on endocrinology, and it stated that one hormone, adrenalin, was
secreted by the adrenal cortex. I mention this to show how
much progress has been made in medicine the past 50 or
60 years in understanding the role the adrenal cortex plays
in the health, or lack of health, of all of us.

Patients suffering from hypoadrenocorticism have feelings of weakness, fatigue, and faintness practically identical with those discussed in the preceding chapter. Dr. Sidney A. Portis reported, after examining many business executives, that hypoglycemia is definitely related to emotional stress. (See *Journal of the American Medical Assoc.*, Dec. 2, 1950). The consensus of those endocrinologists who have made extensive studies of hypoadrenocorticism and emotional instability, is that the emotional instability is functional in nature and directly attributable to the hypofunction or malfunction of the adrenal cortex.

Dr. Tintera has worked out a splendid threefold program for attacking hypoadrenocorticism. He believes that patients are always subject to various stresses, and that they should be told by their doctors how harmful dietary indiscretions, fatigue, worry, and intoxicating liquors are. According to Dr. Tintera, the patients must receive from their physicians complete but simple explanations of the nature of their illnesses; the patients will try to adjust their activities and keep on the prescribed diet more willingly if they understand how emotional upsets can produce the hated symptoms and how excessive eating of carbohydrates can put an end to a period of well-being and bring about a return of weakness and fatigue.

This, briefly stated, is Dr. Tintera's program, as he has explained it in several articles appearing in the medical journals:

1. *Adjustment of the patient's activity*

These patients must be taught to take environmental and emotional stress in stride. Frequently, their ideas and attitudes must be changed. This is no easy thing to do, particularly with older people. As Dr. Tintera states, "This aspect of treatment is most important and probably most difficult to achieve quickly and successfully." Merely to tell patients to take stress in stride and then expect a dramatic result would be either idle or naive.

If we want to change their ideas and attitudes, we must go to a deeper level; we have to inquire about the "why" of their ideas and attitudes. We cannot always believe what they tell us, but we have made the first attempt. Maybe we can get at the motivation—one answer to the "why." Then we may have a look at the familial and economic setting. There will be perhaps a dozen other ways to try to find what we set out to learn about these people.

If we can get them to change their ideas and attitudes, increase the widths of their horizons, experience the adventure of getting out of some of their timeworn grooves —in short, get them to live and to want to live—they will not, at least, be early candidates for senility. As it is, most people are shallow at best.

Many of these people have already worked out routines which help them control their emotions. They will learn quickly that they can avoid hypoglycemic reactions by eating less at meal times and by taking snacks between meals and at bed time. They must all be taught that eating candy or any food with sugar is completely out.

I anticipate that someone who has been reading health fad ads is going to ask: "How about taking raw sugar? Will that do any harm?" The best answer to that question is a statement by Dr. Cora Miller of the Greater Los Angeles

Nutrition Council: "The only thing of importance that white sugar lacks and raw sugar contains is dirt."

2. *Drug therapy*

The primary aim of drug therapy is to put the adrenal cortex at rest temporarily to allow the cells to return to a functioning state so they will subsequently be able to respond normally to stress. Therapy consists of injections of adrenal cortex extract.

These injections, manufactured from the adrenals of young domestic animals, are given frequently at first. As adrenal cortex sufficiency improves, the frequency of the injections is diminished. Ultimately, provided he has cooperated by dieting properly and avoiding undue emotional exertion, the patient will progress satisfactorily without any further injections. Sometimes, however, a periodic checkup may indicate that the injections of the adrenal cortex extract should be temporarily resumed.

Please do not get the idea that you will have to receive these injections for the rest of your life. Whenever your weakened and impaired adrenal glands are put into proper working condition, the drug therapy can be discontinued. No doctor can tell you how long that will take. It may only be a few months or it may be a year or more. As you have already determined from what you have read, the seriousness of the impairment of your adrenals, the control you maintain over your emotions, and the steadfastness with which you stick to the diet, will determine the length of time you will have to take these "shots."

The use of the whole adrenal cortex extract (usually

made from the adrenals of young beef cattle) in the treatment of adrenal disease has been neglected by the medical
profession since the development of cortisone and ACTH. I
am sure the reason is that cortisone and ACTH act much
faster than does the adrenal cortex extract.

The new method of treating allergic conditions as related to an adrenal cortical insufficiency recognizes that
the patient is an ill person who needs to be treated as such
rather than symptomatically. The overall result is not only
relief from allergies, but also an improvement in the
patient's general health. Treatment with the whole adrenal
cortex extract aims at restoring normal bodily functions.
Individual steroids, such as cortisone, hydrocortisone and
the like, give dramatic temporary relief but may pro-
foundly suppress the function of the adrenals in addition
to producing side effects. Such drastic action is not necessary when dietary regimen supports the effect of the
adrenal cortex extract.

Dr. Herbert B. Goldman, a prominent otolaryngologist,
says that knowledge of hormonal dysfunction can be
applied to a considerable number of otolaryngologic conditions, many of which have resisted standard treatment.
I quote from an article by Dr. Goldman appearing in the
American Medical Association Archives of Otolaryngology,
Nov., 1956:

> Application of these endocrinologic principles opens a new
> vista in the relief of these heretofore regarded as unim-
> portant but extremely distressing and aggravating condi-
> tions, so that patients may enjoy the full bounty of normal
> health. These are the patients who would return continu-

ously with the same symptoms despite the nasal tampons
and various throat gargles and sprays and antibiotics. . . .
At times, by the simple expedient of limiting carbohydrates
in children, we have eliminated the distressing symptoms
of nasal stuffiness. Readily absorbable carbohydrates, including alcohol, in any form, act as a definite and violent
stressor agent of the adrenal cortex.

3. Diet

The diet for the hypoadrenocortical state is the same as
that recommended for hypoglycemia and given you in
the previous chapter.

We must not forget that what is attempted in the cure
of hypoadrenocorticism is the restoration of weak, semi-
exhausted adrenals to normal health. The high protein,
medium fat, low carbohydrate diet has been found to
place the least amount of strain on the adrenals. The
adrenal cortex extract injections give the glands a rest
and allow them to recuperate while the hormone supplements look after the body chemistry. Endocrinologists
have known for some time that our adrenal glands will
"beat back" from weakness and sometimes from disease
if given an opportunity to do so.

The purpose of Dr. Tintera's three-point program is,
in summary, to recondition the endocrine glands—particularly the adrenals and the pancreas, with its islands
of Langerhans—to secrete their hormones in sufficient
amounts and proper proportions.

Dr. Tintera says that most allergics have poorly functioning adrenals and that their allergic diseases generally
respond to a treatment which puts the adrenals into proper

working order. He explains why some of us—sensitive to this, that, and the other substance—suffer so much from allergies, while others are not affected sufficiently by any foreign substance to cause any allergic woes: "Endocrinology has now gotten deep below the end results of allergic processes. In learning about the intricate and subtle chemistry of the adrenal glands, it discovered that the difference between the nonallergic majority and the allergic minority was the difference between strong, alertly responsive adrenals which can and do marshal the body's defenses in a flash, and weak, sluggish glands which are incapable of doing what they should."

In order to understand why one man's food is another man's poison, or stated another way, why over 150 million Americans are not made ill by the invaders which make nearly 18 million Americans miserable, and often at least temporarily disabled, we must remember two things:

(1) The central command post of our body's defenses is our adrenals, and,

(2) Body chemistry is exceedingly intolerant of all substances but its own. Foreign substances generally are broken down and converted chemically—animal proteins into human proteins, vegetable carbohydrates into human carbohydrates, and so forth.

Some foreign substances like bacteria have to be killed, or at least prevented from multiplying; otherwise we would die of infections. Other foreign substances have to be neutralized chemically and made harmless. These are the substances which cause allergies if the body chemistry cannot neutralize them.

In most persons, the bodily defenses are adequate in warding off any attack by outside substances; such persons do not suffer from allergies. Without the assistance of the hormones from the adrenal cortices, however, there can be no adequate defense. If the adrenals are underfunctioning, or if they are partially exhausted, they cannot fully respond to stimulation and the essential adrenal cortex hormones they produce are insufficient in amount and chemically out of balance with the rest of the endocrine system.

When grass or weed pollen to which you are sensitive enters through the nostrils or mouth, you have hay fever; when your defense mechanism fails in the bronchial passages, you have asthma; if this happens in the lining of your stomach, you have some kind of food allergy, perhaps hives; if it occurs in the skin, you have a rash or eczema.

On the other hand, if your adrenals are up to par, you will probably never realize that any of these foreign substances invaded your body. If you were born with weak adrenals, in all probability you have suffered from one or more allergic diseases all of your life.

A person with very poor adrenals may live such a sheltered life, free from stress or strain, that he will never have allergic disorders. But who would want to live such a life, even if possible? Without stress or strain we would have little or no pleasure in living.

The hormones from the adrenal cortex prepare the body to withstand stress, and if the adrenals are not strong and healthy at birth, and if they are not strengthened by diet, drugs (such as adrenal cortex extract), and the avoidance of unnecessary stress, the whole body will some-day be in trouble.

Fortunately, most Americans are born with adrenals of apparently super strength. The reason I say this is that the American diet is bad enough to tear down adrenals with any degree of weakness. The amazing thing is how the most perfect adrenal glands withstand the onslaught of the common American diet.

Many of us drink ten or fifteen cups of coffee daily. Our meals are loaded with sugar and starches. We drink sugared cola drinks loaded with caffeine between meals. If we attend an evening meeting of any kind, there are the inevitable coffee and sweets of some type.

Did you ever observe what the ladies serve when they get together for a meeting? Most of them will be talking about how hard they have been dieting to take off some pounds, yet the food served will be rich in calories from sugar, starch, and fat, and everyone will be expected to drink more than one cup of coffee.

Go to your school cafeteria and see what your youngsters are eating and drinking. Sugars and other quickly absorbed carbohydrates often constitute the main part of their noon-day meals. The handy dispensing machines for punchasing sweetened drinks, including cola, frequently furnish our children with more liquid than do the cold water fountains.

I was pleased to read the following statement from the *American Medical Association's Council on Food and Nutrition*, issued June 30, 1962:

> Every effort should be expended to encourage students to adopt and enjoy good food habits.

The availability of confections and carbonated beverages on school premises may tempt children to spend lunch money for them and lead to poor food habits. Their high energy value and continual availability are likely to affect children's appetites for regular meals.

Expenditures for carbonated beverages and most confections yield a nutritional return greatly inferior to that of milk, fruit and other foods included in the basic food groups.

In view of these considerations, the council is particularly opposed to sale and distribution of confections and carbonated beverages in school lunch rooms.

The endocrinologists tell us that the hormones from our adrenal cortices and the hormones from the medulla are so important that without them life is impossible. The adrenal hormones regulate the chemical conversion of food into fuel and building materials. They regulate the transportation of fuel throughout the body for "burning" with oxygen in each and every tissue, and the transport of the building materials and its uses in repairing and replacing cells and tissues.

The greatest break for allergy sufferers, with their weak and poorly functioning adrenals, is the established medical fact that the adrenal glands have recuperative power. Without this, the millions who have known the agonies, and sometimes the despair, of allergic diseases would have little hope of a better tomorrow.

Should one ever attempt to cure his allergies by dieting and taking the adrenal cortex extract injections without first seeing a physician for an examination and tests? The answer is a definite and emphatic No. However, you will find the examination and tests are not as complicated and expensive as you may have anticipated. Most doctors who treat allergic patients by diet and the glandular therapy require a thorough endocrine history and a physical examination before making tests, which consist of a glucose tolerance test, a complete blood count, a protein bound iodine test, and a urine analysis.

Some physicians, so I am told, insist on a more elaborate series of laboratory tests to determine the status of the adrenal function. Generally, however, doctors say the minimal testing shown above is thoroughly adequate for detecting any dysfunction.

Not all doctors use the same glucose tolerance test. A six hour or a four hour oral glucose tolerance test is perhaps more widely used than any other.

As far as I know, no doctor permits his patients to drink coffee while following the diet and getting the adrenal cortex extracts. Physicians, however, are not agreed on the necessity of excluding tobacco during such time. I believe I can safely say all of them agree that no patient should smoke early in the morning before breakfast and that smoking should be kept in moderate bounds. Some doctors forbid smoking altogether, others discourage smoking, particularly excessive smoking, and others permit a moderate amount of smoking.

You may ask if it is necessary to take the injections. Is adrenal cortex extract available in a form which can be taken orally? Yes, there are commercial preparations manufactured by reliable pharmaceutical companies on the market. About a year ago, before I went off coffee a second time, I took several bottles of tablets of adrenal cortex extract. I did not find them very effective, however, and they are more expensive than the injections. I think the reason the tablets did not help me as much as the injections did is that adrenal cortex extract is composed of hormones; like the insulin given orally to diabetics, it is, in the oral form, at least partially digested in the stomach and intestinal tracts.

It is my opinion that when our doctors and the general public awake to the necessity for every allergic victim to be tested for hypoadrenocorticism, there will come, out of the research centers somewhere in America, the discovery of a drug that can be taken by mouth and have the same efficiency as the adrenal cortex extract injections. Undoubtedly, too, such a drug will be sold at a fraction of the present cost of the inefficient oral preparations available today. I do not believe this is merely wishful thinking on my part.

5.

YOU CAN'T
ARGUE AGAINST SUCCESS

Before I heard that allergies were being cured by diet and adrenal cortex extract, six wholly unrelated incidents convinced me that my adrenal glands were in some way involved in all of the many allergic diseases from which I have suffered. These are, in the order of their happening:

1. In 1921, I was present when a business establishment was robbed by a masked bandit and later the same year I happened to be on a public street in close proximity to a gunfight between police officers and some men who had just committed a robbery. Three men were killed in the battle of bullets. To say that I was frightened on both occasions is a gross understatement. After each incident, I observed my usually stopped-up nose was open and my breathing was free and easy. A doctor's explanation of why the breathing through my nose and mouth was so much easier than usual was that the fright caused my adrenal glands to be overactive for the time being. What happened

beyond that he said he had no way of knowing; evidently it was due to some kind of body chemistry which he admitted he did not understand.

2. I have already mentioned the adrenalin kit I was given by an allergist in the early thirties and told to use when I had breathing difficulties.

3. In 1939, there was a lot of publicity about a vitamin, pantothenic acid, which was supposed to stop hair from becoming gray. Like many other vain people, I purchased a bottle of these tablets, hoping they would prevent my hair from changing its color. I discovered that the vitamin tablets caused me to feel considerably better than I had felt before taking them.

I wrote a letter to the manufacturer of the product, a reliable pharmaceutical house, and asked for an explanation for the favorable effect. I received a long letter from the company, stating, among other things, that pantothenic acid is involved in adrenal function. The letter quoted some doctor as having referred to the close correlation of this particular vitamin with the adrenal cortex.

4. In 1940, I went on a candy bar spree one evening, eating at least a dozen candy bars loaded with sugar. The next morning I had a hangover, exactly as if I had been grossly intoxicated the night before, even though I had taken no liquor of any kind. I had a terrible headache; I was weak, shaky, and nervous. I went to a doctor and told him what I had done and how I felt. He remarked: "If you had taken enough liquor to put you in that shape I would have given you a shot of adrenal cortex extract. All I can do, however, is to tell you to go home and to bed and

lay off the sugar." I asked the doctor if this drug he talked about was harmful. He assured me it was perfectly harmless, but said its effect on allergics was not known. When I begged him to give me some of the adrenal cortex extract, he told me again that he didn't think it would do me any good and that it was expensive. I insisted on taking the maximum dosage, 10 cc., intravenously. In order to get rid of me, I suppose, he gave me the injection—all the contents of a small glass vial. Within a few hours I was over my hangover and felt fine. When I reported this to the doctor, he said he was astonished that the extract had worked so well and so quickly. I am not certain he believed me when I told him it was an overload of candy that had knocked me out.

5. In 1957, I took a vacation trip in the New England states. Before starting east, I packed a large bottle of antihistamine tablets, since I knew I would be eating shell seafoods nearly every day. This medication may have helped during the early part of the trip, but about the time I was ready to fly home, my eyes were nearly swollen shut. The first thing I did when I got back to Oklahoma was to go to a doctor. Before I could tell him about my troubles, he observed that I had about the worst case of skin allergy he had ever seen. I told him how ineffective my antihistamines had been. He asked how much of my body was so affected and, after an examination of my itching body, remarked: "Cortisone is to be used in allergy cases only in emergencies. If this isn't an emergency, I never saw one. This prescription calls for 16 tablets. Take four a day and you should be over your skin condition in four days. The

tablets will cost you fifty cents each. Go right ahead with your antihistamines; there will be no conflict with the cortisone."

At the end of the four days, my skin allergy was gone and I felt great. I said, "This is it; it's expensive, but it's worth it to stop these allergic attacks." I had at last found the end of the rainbow for which I had been looking for so many years. My enthusiasm for my new remedy, cortisone, was short-lived, however, for I soon learned from the doctors that the cure was worse than the disease.

At last I had definitely established to my satisfaction that one hormone from the adrenal glands, cortisone, could and would put an end to a severe allergic attack when everything else failed. Where I went from there I had not the slightest idea, but I had the feeling I wasn't far from the cure for allergies. How right I was!

6. In 1958, I inadvertently overlooked paying a disability premium on a United States government life insurance policy. The disability clause provided that after I became 65 no more premiums would be required. As soon as they received my application for reinstatement, the Veterans Administration wrote me that since only one more annual premium would be due on the disability clause, I would have to go to a Veterans Administration hospital for a physical examination. A day for the examination was suggested, which I immediately accepted.

At this hospital I was given a fairly thorough examination. One of the doctors stated to me: "Your blood pressure is way too low. Have you ever been treated for Addison's disease?" I informed him I had not. I then asked: "Doctor what is the significance of my low blood pressure?" He remarked that low blood pressure readings were usually indicative of decreased chemical activity within the body. "In your case," he said, "I would imagine the adrenal glands are involved."

In March, 1959, Dr. J. Wendall Mercer, our family physician and a general practitioner, put me on the diet and medication for hypoadrenocorticism. I can truthfully say I enjoyed the diet from the first day, and the only complaint I had was about the headaches I suffered after I eliminated coffee. When one has been a heavy coffee drinker for 50 years, he should not expect to get over the effects of the caffeine immediately. It was about two weeks before I adjusted to being without coffee.

For one week, I had an adrenal cortex extract injection each day. For the next three weeks, I got the shots three times each week, and then, for about three months, twice each week. After that, I got only a shot each week until the end of nine months, at which time I got a shot every other week until the end of one year, or March, 1960.

At that time, I told Dr. Mercer I believed I was cured and would discontinue the injections and the diet. He advised against doing so. His statement was: "You had allergies a long time before you started this program. You admit you like the diet, and you have never had a sore arm from the injections. Why don't you continue for another year? You have had most of your expense this first year. We will try giving you the shots every four weeks and see how you get along."

I continued the treatment for another year, getting the

shots once every month. In March, 1961, I discontinued
the diet and the drugs and, with the exception of the time
I tried to use the oral adrenal cortex extract, I have not
taken adrenal cortex extract since. However, I did have
some difficulties with my diet, as I shall later explain.

A man in his middle or upper sixties never tires of hearing how well he looks, especially if he can construe the
words as meaning he looks younger. When I made a routine
round of the counties in my judicial district in May, 1959,
the lawyers, clerks, and other court officials remarked how
well I looked and inquired if I had been on vacation. I
was enjoying such a wonderful state of health, with no
allergies so soon after I began the treatment, that I am
sure I bored everyone who would listen to me with my
enthusiastic report on the progress I was making.

From March, 1959, to March, 1961, I eliminated every
food to which I knew I was sensitive, including milk. A
dentist had told me bone meal is an excellent substitute
for milk in providing minerals; other dentists agreed that
bone meal might safely be substituted for milk as a bone
and teeth builder.

For two years I took six plain bone meal tablets daily,
and I have conclusive proof that bone meal is a good source
of minerals. Early in 1959, I was in an automobile accident in which my legs were injured. My doctors told me
at that time that the X-ray films showed a marked calcium
deficiency in both legs. In the summer of 1961, my legs
were again X-rayed and the films indicated a normal
supply of bone calcium.

The same ophthalmologist has regularly examined my

eyes and fitted my glasses for the past 35 years. Since I reached the age of 50, the lenses in my glasses had been changed about every two years until 1961, when I went to this doctor for a routine checkup of my eyes. He seemed to spend more time than usual making his examinations. Finally he said, "This is incredible. When I examined you a little over two years ago, you had a mild case of arteriosclerosis. Now you show only a trace of hardening of the arteries. What have you done to make that change?"

I told the doctor about the diet and the medication I had been on for two years to cure my allergies. He said he had noticed how well I looked when he first saw me that day. "You are the first patient I've had who has taken adrenal cortex extract and a special diet over an extended period of time. Your health seems to be excellent. By the way, I can't improve on the glasses you are wearing," were his remarks.

The lenses in the glasses I am now wearing, fitted late in 1958, were found satisfactory by another examination in 1963. I always have two sets of glasses fitted at each change, one for general use and a tinted one for driving. My saving on glasses since March, 1959, has been more than a hundred dollars.

Other physicians who have examined me since March, 1961, report that I am in excellent physical condition. My blood pressure since 1960 has remained about the same and, according to the doctors, is as near perfect for my age as is possible.

While on the treatment, I started exercising regularly. At first a mile walk was about my limit. Now I try to do three or four miles of walking along with other vigorous exercises each day when the weather permits. I find I can take a five mile hike with less fatigue than when I was forty.

In 1959, my weight went down to where it was when I was 30 years old, without any effort on my part to reduce. It has remained constant since 1959, except for a part of 1961 and 1962. After I went off the diet in March, 1961, I soon began to gain weight; in fact, by the end of 1961 I once again weighed what I did early in 1959. I then resumed, in the main, the high protein, low carbohydrate diet, and it wasn't long until I again weighed the same as I did when I was thirty. I intend to remain on the high protein, low carbohydrate diet for the remainder of my life, since I know it is best for me.

However, at all times since I discontinued the diet in March, 1961, I have paid no attention to allergic or nonallergic foods. I still prefer the powdered nonfat milk which I traded for the bone meal tablets in 1961. I had no tobacco problem, because I had stopped smoking before 1959. I have for many years been a teetotaler, so I had no adjustments to make to liquor before or after the treatments.

I have about the same enthusiasm for my judicial work as I had the first year I was on the bench. One strange fact is that I find that everyone I deal with appears to be a much finer person than he was in January or February, 1959. According to what the lawyers say, I am now a much easier judge to try a case before than I was in 1958 and before. It never occurred to me, until the last few years, that a relaxed judge means relaxed lawyers, litigants, witnesses, jurors, bailiffs, clerks, reporters, and other officials, and even relaxed spectators.

After I had good health and my previous symptoms of allergy had been alleviated, I discussed my case with four doctors, all friends of mine. None of them had ever treated me, and their reactions to my enthusiastic report of what had happened were most pessimistic.

Dr. A. said he would not want a patient of his to have "all that steroid injected into his body."

Dr. B. responded by saying, "You patients build up a lot of psychological momentum over something new and fantastic, but it won't last."

Dr. C. stated his patients couldn't afford such luxurious foods and drugs.

Dr. D. indicated he would go along with those specially trained in allergies until they changed their minds about what methods they would use.

Why did all four of these excellent physicians take such a defensive attitude? I had not accused them of doing anything wrong. Was it because I, a layman, may have expressed a medical opinion? Was it because they believed a layman is always wrong in his opinions about his own physical condition? It couldn't be because doctors are always right. As a trial judge, I have gotten so used to hearing certain doctors testify for complainants in damage suits and certain other well-known insurance company doctors testify for the parties sued, that I frequently know in advance, from reading the pleadings in the cases, approximately what each doctor is going to tell the court and jury.

You may be ready to ask me how many others have benefited from this comparatively new way of doing something for allergy sufferers. I can't answer that question accurately because, as a layman, I cannot get facts and figures from physicians. I know the number cured is large and the per cent of failures is small. Dr. Mercer told me that he had the same dramatic results with other allergic patients who went on the diet and took the shots as he had with me. Dr. Tintera, in a very recent medical article, stated: "I have treated hundreds of cases with a very small percentage of failures. The failures have been due primarily to more serious underlying conditions such as emphysema or fibrosis of the lungs, or in patients who have been previously subjected to intensive cortisone therapy."

It is easy for me to understand the doctors' conservatism because I belong to a profession that is more conservative than theirs. Lawyers generally are opposed to any changes in practice or procedure. They remind me of the old man who lived 50 years on the farm his father homesteaded 100 years before. A tourist stopped at the farm to make some inquiry and, after learning how long the man had resided there, remarked, "You must have seen many changes in your nation, state, and community in the past 50 years." The old gentleman answered, "Yes, I have; and I have been against all of them."

It is only natural that some physicians express opposition to any plan of treating allergies different from the one employed by the allergists for nearly half a century.

Even if every patient who received the adrenal cortex extract and followed the antihypoglycemia diet were to experience complete recovery from all allergic diseases, some reactionary doctors would brand the method of treatment as unorthodox, unconventional and unsafe until more was known about it. I read somewhere that penicillin was not accepted generally by the medical profession until nearly twenty-five years after it was discovered.

The important thing to keep in mind is that there are no records of any patient having suffered any adverse effects from the use of the whole adrenal cortex extract. Those doctors who have not approved this method of treating allergies do not contend it can or will have any harmful effect. Their objections are based on grounds other than injury to a patient.

Many persons who were lifelong allergy sufferers heard about my recovery and sought information from me. The first question each one asked was "Can the treatments do me any harm?" I assured all of them there would be no adverse effects and strongly urged them to do as I had done. I insisted that they first take tests to ascertain if they had hypoadrenocorticism and that they do nothing until a physician advised that the diet would not be injurious and that need for adrenal cortex extract was indicated. I urged them to try this new and successful method of treatment if their doctors told them they might safely do so. "You have nothing to lose but your allergies and your wretched health," was always my final argument to each one who inquired.

All of those who came to me for a word of hope belonged to that great unnamed fraternity of men and women who from time to time have said to each other, between sneezes, wheezes, noseblowings, coughing, spitting, scratching, and yawning, "You ought to go see my doctor. He cured me." A few of them were bitter toward all doctors, but most of them were just hanging on, hoping some miracle would happen so they could enjoy life as other people do. Not one of them reported even a partial failure of the hypoadrenocorticism treatments, and every letter and telephone call I got from them was a glowing tribute to the efficacy of the treatments.

Returning to the objections of some doctors to the hypoadrenocorticism treatment of allergies, let us examine their principal objections and see how much merit, if any, there is in what they say.

1. Some of my inquirers have reported back to me that their doctors said the treatment was not one generally accepted by the medical profession. To make such a statement is, of course, to say the obvious. I dare say nearly every routine treatment employed daily in a doctor's office was not, at one time, generally accepted by the medical profession. We don't have to confine our remarks to medicine to know that most of our everyday actions haven't always been accepted as the most effective way of doing things. This objection, if we dignify it by calling it that, is too absurd to discuss further.

2. A few doctors, so I hear, claim adrenal cortex extract has only "historical value," whatever that means. These doubting Thomases should read the medical histories of thousands upon thousands of allergics, who, after

trying everything recommended to them by their doctors, despaired of ever having good health until they found this new and phenomenal way to relief. These histories will provide something of "historical value" to the medical profession now and in the years to come.

If we assume these doctors mean that proponents of the adrenocorticism method of treatment must produce statistics showing how many dogs, cats, rabbits, mice, and the like have responded favorably to adrenal cortex extract in allergy cases, their position is preposterous. As Dr. E. M. Abrahamson so aptly pointed out, man is the only animal known to suffer from allergies.

These "historical value" physicians daily prescribe cortisone, ACTH, and other steroid compounds, knowing the danger that can and will result therefrom. They know that adrenal cortex extract will never cause any bad side effects.

3. Some doctors bitterly object to the term "subclinical Addison's disease" used by certain specialists who have had close to one hundred per cent success in the treatment of chronic allergy cases—patients who had been discarded by reputable physicians and frequently found their way into the clutches of unscrupulous practitioners before they were told about the new way of curing allergies.

To the layman's way of thinking, it makes no difference whether these people were or were not suffering from "subclinical Addison's disease." The only thing of importance to the patient is that he got relief from his suffering. I go along with the doctors who call the condition of these distressed people "subclinical Addison's disease" solely because they were right and other doctors were wrong in alleviating my symptoms.

4. Physicians have objected to the cost of the treatments. It is true that adrenal cortex extract is expensive, and a high protein diet costs more than one loaded with bread, potatoes, rice, and pies or cakes.

It would seem that the patients instead of the doctors should be the ones to complain about costs. Over a long period of years, an allergic patient will spend a lot of money for medical and drug bills and still be seeking relief. If the patient recovers his health, or improves it by means of the diet and injections, the medical and food expenses may well be, in the long run, the cheapest medication and food costs the patient ever had.

Before a doctor becomes too upset about what his patient is going to have to spend for food and adrenal cortex extract, I suggest he turn the picture around and have a look at what he may see on the other side. I am talking about a young or middle-aged wage earner whose only source of income is what he makes with his head and his hands, a worker with excellent earning capacity, but unable to keep a good job because of lack of health. Is this treatment too expensive for such a person? Should he be disposed of by having his cards at the employment agencies marked "Irascible and undesirable," or should he be given treatments, even if expensive? This man is not looking for handouts for himself and his family. Almost every one of these people has a sense of dignity and a respect for the rights and properties of others, regardless of how poverty stricken he may have become as a result of his inability to get and hold a job because of his allergic diseases.

Do I consider my recovery too expensive? I'll let you be the judge of that. Excepting the expenses incurred by surgery and an automobile accident in 1959, I have spent less for medical treatment and drugs from 1959 to 1963, both inclusive, than in any five year period since 1931. The entire cost of the adrenal cortex therapy in 1959 and 1960 was less than the average total cost of one major operation performed every day in practically every hospital in the nation. My proof for this statement comes from figures released by national and state hospital associations.

Before I went on this treatment, I worried most of the time whether I would be able to continue holding a state judicial office. My future problem will be to decide how much longer I want to remain an active trial judge.

As I shall later show, there are innumerable ways to lower the costs of a high protein diet. We live well, and our grocery bills are no higher than those of our friends whose incomes are comparable to ours. Regardless of how much some doctors may want to sympathize with me about the cost of adrenal cortex extract and good food, I can't put a price tag on the value of my good health.

In the damage suits brought to my courts, juries and I, as the trial judge, try to determine in dollars the value of good health to one who has lost it by the negligence of another. What is the monetary value of good health? Would you say five thousand dollars, ten thousand dollars, twenty-five thousand dollars, a hundred thousand dollars, or even more?

While some doctor is fuming about the high cost of adrenal cortex extract and high protein foods, another doctor—maybe the family physician who helped bring the patient or his children into the world—is getting tremendous pleasure from helping his patient regain health and strength and take his rightful place in society. Which of these physicians do you believe is the wiser?

6.

A DIET YOU WILL LIKE

I KNOW THAT most people, especially men, object to any kind of diet. I also know that many women have unsuccessfully been on a myriad of diets, trying to get back their youthful figures. Nearly all articles on reducing either start or conclude with the statement that obese persons eat more than their bodies require; that reduction of daily caloric consumption is the only way to reduce. Short term crash diets are starvation diets. Prepared liquid reducing foods are generally too high in carbohydrates to have much reducing value.

Calories do count when it comes to gaining or losing weight. Measuring and weighing every food item to get a certain number of calories is distasteful to most of us. The antihypoglycemia diet is low in calories, high in nutritional value, and can readily be adjusted to your bodily needs. What I mean is this: If you want to take off weight, instead of counting calories, take smaller servings of the fats and eat those foods having a lower percentage of carbohydrates.

If you are eating every food permitted but are not reducing, I suggest that you try the foods that are not more than fifteen per cent carbohydrate. If you continue to gain weight, I recommend that you eat foods with not more than ten per cent carbohydrate content. If it is essential for you to lose weight, you can—for a limited time—eat no foods containing more than six per cent carbohydrate and limit the amount of your protein foods. I can take off weight easily and quickly by cutting down on my carbohydrates; that I have never eaten less protein and salad foods while reducing, accounts for my never having been abnormally hungry since I started the diet in 1959.

Once you get your weight where you want it you can start increasing the percentage of the carbohydrates. You will soon find how easy it is to keep your weight the same without that half-starved feeling with which you are so familiar.

A disadvantage of starvation diets is that one who has been on one of them looks older after he has lost weight. If you follow the antihypoglycemia diet, however, you will look younger as the pounds melt away.

Please do not get the impression that this diet was worked out for weight reducers. It is aimed at improving the function of the endocrines—particularly the adrenals and the pancreas, with its islands of Langerhans. However, it is a wonderful reducing diet.

One benefit of the diet and the adrenal cortex medication is that they slow down the course of degenerative diseases that normally come with the years, arteriosclerosis and many others. My own experiences with the diet and drug injections convinced me that getting old is largely

the result of malnutrition. Doctors tell us that most people
who have aged prematurely have been starved of vitamins
and minerals. Often, these doctors say, it is difficult to
pinpoint the direct cause of malnutrition since the subjects are subclinical cases rather than the classical textbook examples of malnutrition.

Medical science has a long way to go in the field of
biochemistry. Dr. Sam E. Roberts of the University of
Kansas Medical School says, in his book *Ear, Nose and
Throat Dysfunctions Due to Deficiencies and Imbalances:*
"The medical students of the past who are our physicians
today were taught little or nothing of nutrition and even
less of deficiencies and imbalances. The authors of *Therapeutic Nutrition* remark that medical school curricula are
preoccupied with diagnosis and specific therapy. Little
time and attention is given to the nutritional aspect of
therapeutics." Dr. Roberts goes on to point out that although biochemistry is taught today, it is taught without
any clinical application or understanding. Dr. Roberts'
views are approved in a foreword to the book by Dr.
Morris Fishbein, whose name is a household word in
American medicine.

You may be a little frightened at the prospect of having
foods to which you are accustomed eliminated from your
diet, but there is no occasion for alarm. It did not take
me long to turn my attention from the bakeries and sweet
shops to the dietetic counters and low calorie sections of
grocery stores and supermarkets. You will be surprised at
what you find in these stores. The artificially sweetened
syrups, jellies, and preserves are as tasty as those you have

been eating. Every kind of canned fruit is available without sugar. The diet includes nearly all fresh fruits, and only a few vegetables arc not permitted.

When fresh fruit is not available I buy water-packed fruit in gallon cans and sweeten it with artificial liquid sweetener which I buy in large bottles and often on sale. Unsweetened canned fruits do not cost as much as those to which sugar has been added. Every nutritional expert says, also, that low priced meats have as much nutritional value as high priced cuts.

Occasionally you may eat a small waffle or hot cake made from gluten and/or soybean flour, using, of course, artificially sweetened syrup or jelly. At one time I made a list of over 100 different desserts which could be included on the diet. If one feels he must eat ice cream, he may have small servings of dietetic (sugarless) ice cream. The low-calorie gelatin desserts which are prepared without sugar are delicious and inexpensive, and sugarless bottled or canned drinks are as good and about the same price as sweetened soft drinks. Each morning I look forward to my two cups of decaffeinated coffee with as much enthusiasm as I formerly had for regular coffee.

Therc are many things we should keep in mind about why we are on this diet and what we hope to accomplish with it. We take snacks between meals and before bedtime, when it is necessary to keep our blood sugar from falling. If we eat three fairly good meals and no more during a day there will be three upward and three downward swings of the blood sugar level, but if we eat less at meal times, and oftener, then there will be six or seven small up and down swings.

When we eat sugar, candy, honey, ice cream, pie, cake, or any quickly absorbed carbohydrate, the sudden rise in blood sugar level stimulates the islets of the pancreas to produce more insulin. The insulin, in turn, gets rid of too much blood sugar and lowers the blood sugar level. This sudden drop is what makes us feel so terrible, and generally starts some kind of allergic attack. An emotional upset also causes the islets of the pancreas to produce more insulin. Therefore, we only eat carbohydrates that are absorbed slowly, and we avoid any stress that causes a sudden drop in blood sugar level. You may have no more breakfasts of coffee and doughnuts or sweet rolls while you are on the diet.

There are many ways the cost of the diet may be kept down. Instant nonfat powdered milk is cheaper than regular milk and just as nutritious. You can eliminate milk and take plain bone meal tablets at a cost of only a few cents a day. Nutritional experts generally recommend that a patient should not drink more than one quart of milk daily to avoid the danger of developing calcium stones in the kidney or bladder. If cheese or cream is used, the milk supply should be reduced accordingly. A pint of milk a day, or its equivalent in other calcium and phosphorus foods, is ordinarily adequate for an adult. Some doctors say that a larger amount of vitamin D than is needed, combined with more than a normal amount of milk, may cause calcium stones.

Doctors recommend increasing the amount of water

intake in order to prevent the formation of calcium stones. They tell us that normally our kidneys excrete any excess of blood calcium if we have an adequate supply of liquids daily.

We should remember that we eat foods to furnish the materials for growth and repair, to provide energy for our work and the functional activities of the organs and tissues of the body, and to maintain body temperature. There is no hard and fast rule as to what part of your diet should be carbohydrate and what part protein.

An inverse ratio exists throughout the world between carbohydrate consumption and income. In America, carbohydrates are normally expected to meet roughly 50 per cent of the total energy requirements. In the tropics and in some impoverished parts of the world, carbohydrates contribute up to 80 per cent of the daily caloric needs.

Roughly speaking, carbohydrates should not furnish more than one third of the hypoglycemic's daily caloric energy. Ordinarily, the antihypoglycemia diet furnishes an adequate supply of vitamins and minerals. Enough fat must be taken to supply the essential fatty acids and fat soluble vitamins. The diet will always provide a sufficient amount of proteins for the work of the defense mechanisms, for tissue repair and maintenance, and for growth, since there is practically no limit on the protein foods allowed.

We must not forget that protein and fat supply potential glucose, which is made available very gradually through metabolic processes. It is best to have our largest protein meal in the evening. Although breakfast is the most important meal of the day, it is essential to have a high protein meal in the evening, since the glucose produced gradually from the protein foods is instrumental in preventing hypoglycemia at night or early in the morning. If we eat an evening meal of quickly absorbed carbohydrates, insulin destroys so much of our blood sugar by or before midnight that we have headaches and an "all in" feeling, and we develop hay fever, asthma, or some other allergic symptom by morning.

Whenever I eat a large steak for dinner I always take a bedtime snack of some slowly absorbed carbohydrate food (generally fruit) to prevent insulin induced hypoglycemia during the night.

Most of us grew up with the belief that we had to eat some sugar every day. This view still persists with many people even though the theory that we need sugar in our diets was exploded years ago. More and more doctors are coming to the conclusion that nobody needs sugar, although persons with normal blood sugar generally are able to eat a reasonable amount of sugar with no harmful effects.

Both saccharin and the cyclamates (sodium cyclamate for those who may have salt and calcium cyclamate for those who may not, or whose salt intake is limited) have long been used by diabetics and are usually harmless. They are inexpensive compounds and have no calories, and you will find them as delicious as cane or beet sugar. Some persons, however, have told me that they are allergic to one or more of the artificial sweeteners and that they break out in a skin rash or skin irritation after a long period of use. I don't believe this is a common complaint of users of either saccharin or cyclamates, but if an allergy should appear, it would be advisable to discontinue use until you determine whether the sweetener is the cause of the allergic condition.

There are three fallacies about older people you should know:

1. *As one grows older, he should become heavier.* Most older persons gain weight as the years pass, although it was not nature's intention. We overeat, eat the wrong kinds of foods, and don't exercise enough. Weight should not increase with the years. The insurance companies' physicians say we should weigh approximately the same at 26 and 62.

2. *We should discontinue exercising as we grow older.* Of course an inactive old man or old woman should not go out and do some violent exercising that will bring on a heart attack. Physicians generally agree, however, that there is as much need for a 70-year-old person to take some reasonable exercise each day if he is to remain strong and healthy, as there is for a ten-year-old child to run and play.

3. *Older people should not eat much.* There is no difference in the mineral and vitamin requirements of the young and the old. The bones of many older people are very fragile. Formerly, doctors thought that demineralization of the bones was caused by a low calcium diet, but now they are confident that it is the result of several additional factors, such as (1) reduced secretion of hormones, (2) reduced absorption of food through the intestines due to

malabsorption, (3) reduced intake of vitamin D, and, for the most part, (4) an inadequate protein diet. Many older people are strongly prejudiced against drinking milk and eating foods high in protein content.

The generally accepted diet for those in their later years is one high in proteins, rich in vitamins and minerals, moderately low in carbohydrates, and low in fats. Oldsters should be required to drink a generous amount of liquids throughout the day—water, milk, coffee and tea when permitted, and fruit juices.

Our older citizens do not look on changes with much favor. Changes usually have to come gradually and with some carefully planned persuasion. When an old man or woman refuses to drink milk, the easiest way to introduce minerals into the diet is by mixing dried nonfat milk in a soup or other food at meal time. If milk in any form is refused, the person may be prevailed upon to take plain bone meal tablets. Sometimes it really takes a diplomat to get an old man or an old woman to accept the foods he or she should eat.

One of the comparatively new developments in food technology is the enrichment and fortification of refined or compounded and processed foods with specific minerals or vitamins. Enrichment and fortification has become accepted routine procedure in the preparation of many popular foods.

Also, since World War II, many foods have been dehydrated to prevent spoilage; the process is safe and involves little or no loss in vitamins and minerals. Persons who cannot eat the fresh products can sometimes tolerate

dried milk and dried eggs. Canning, freezing and refriger-
ation arc othcr major methods of food preservation. Fruits
and vegetables canned within 24 hours of picking have
higher vitamin content than fresh fruits and vegetables
bought on the open market after prolonged shippiug aud
storage.

Glycogen (the form in which the liver stores carbohydrates) is also found in small quantities in practically
all other organs of the body. The skeletal, cardiac, and
smooth muscles maintain their own glycogen stores when
at rest or under minor work loads. The conversion of
glucose into glycogen is reversible; when quick absorbtion
of carbohydrates (especially glucose) raises the blood
sugar level, the tide is counteracted by glycogenesis in
the liver and withdrawal of glucose from circulation by
body tissues for the purposes of energy metabolism and
storage against future needs. Glycogenesis has been defined as the conversion of glycogen into glucose or the
conversion of glucose into glycogen. (See Webster's In-
ternational Dictionary and Stedman's Medical Dictionary.)

Despite the continual danger warnings in the news-
papers, magazines, and other news media, more than 20
per cent of all adults are overweight to the extent that
health may be impaired. We are told that obesity aggra-
vates cardiovascular disease and osteoarthritis. It may
cause hypertension, atherosclerosis, hernia, and gall-
bladder disease. In predisposed persons, it may bring on
diabetes. It makes surgery more hazardous, causes postural
derangement, and makes a person appear older than he

actually is. Mortality from most diseases is much higher among the obese.

Unfortunately, the obese have been victimized by many products advertised as harmless weight reducers. All sorts of pharmaceutical preparations are available and sometimes sold without prescriptions. These include appetite depressants, substances which increase the basal metabolism rate, and metabolized vegetable gums. Few physicians regard these as desirable aids in reducing weight.

When I started the diet and the medication in 1959, I had one purpose in mind—to alleviate my allergic diseases. When I discovered that the diet was wonderful for reducing and obtaining good health, you can understand how jubilant I was. My enthusiasm for and my belief in the antihypoglycemia diet and adrenal cortex extract medication are unbounded. With this treatment one may achieve what he dreams about, but never expects to experience—he may find relief from allergic diseases, regain good health, return to a trim and youthful figure, attain emotional stability, and slow down the degenerative diseases that go with age.

If your tests and physical examination indicate that this new treatment might help you, all I ask is that you give it a fair and reasonable trial. It won't be long before you can tell whether it will do for you what it did for me. If it doesn't work with you after a reasonable time, drop it. No harm will have been done and it won't be the first money you have spent on something recommended to you without beneficial results.

If and when you go on the diet, use your imagination

and curiosity in selecting your meals and snacks. There is no more reason for you to be bored by monotony than there was before you started the treatment. There are so many, many foods you are permitted to eat.

I repeat, it is imperative that you stay on the diet every day. If you eat out you will have no difficulties, since restaurants will gladly make substitutions for the starchy vegetables that come with regular meals. Most waitresses will assume that you are a diabetic and do their best to obtain foods you can eat. Cafeterias will be your best bet for getting what you want and may eat.

The practice of saying No to offers of coffee, sweets, and other forbidden foods when you attend parties, committee meetings, teas, after-meeting refreshment periods and the like, will become a valuable habit when rich desserts are offered you, even after you leave the diet.

The diet will appeal to women because they are natural shoppers. I have always hated shopping, but I enjoy going through grocery stores, supermarkets, department stores, drug stores, and health food stores, looking for sugar-free and low carbohydrate foods, which I find in abundance. If you are not accustomed to so doing, you will soon learn to read what is on the printed labels of canned foods to find out the sugar and other carbohydrate contents.

SUGGESTED INEXPENSIVE MENU

On arising in the morning
Fruit juice not sweetened with sugar

Breakfast

One thin slice toasted protein bread with butter
or margarine and dietetic jelly
Fresh fruit or canned fruit artificially sweetened
One egg; boiled, poached, scrambled or fried
Decaffeinated coffee

Mid-morning snack

Cheese (any kind) with 2 or 3 saltines

Lunch

Egg and cheese sandwich (open face) made with one
slice of toasted protein bread; butter or
margarine (not corn) optional
Sliced tomatoes
Serving of cooked vegetable
Molded gelatin dessert with or without artificially
sweetened mixed fruits
Milk or bone meal tablets

Mid-afternoon snack

Salted nuts or dietetic peanut butter rolled up
in a leaf of lettuce

Dinner

Mixed green vegetable salad with small amount of
French or mayonnaise dressing
Hamburger steak
Serving of cooked vegetable
Any permitted fruit for dessert
Decaffeinated coffee

Bedtime snack

Glass of milk and one thin slice of protein bread
or 2 or 3 saltines

SUGGESTED MENU—MORE EXPENSIVE

On arising in the morning

Fruit juice not sweetened with sugar

Breakfast

Ham or sausage and one egg
One thin slice protein bread, toasted if desired,
with butter or margarine
Fruit, such as half grapefruit, orange, non-
sweetened apple sauce, or any other fruit
not excluded from diet
Decaffeinated coffee

Mid-morning snack

Milk or dietetic peanut butter and 2 or 3 saltines

Lunch

Grated carrot and cabbage or lettuce salad
Chicken or fish
Cooked vegetable
One slice of protein bread (toasted if desired)
with butter or margarine
Melon, any kind

Mid-afternoon snack

Salted nuts

Dinner

Cottage cheese salad
Pork chops or lamb chops
Cooked vegetable
Cooked dried fruit or fresh fruit
Decaffeinated coffee

Bedtime snack

Glass of milk and some permitted fruit

SUGGESTED MENU—MORE EXPENSIVE

On arising in the morning

Fruit juice not sweetened with sugar

Breakfast

Bacon and two eggs
One thin slice protein bread (may be toasted)
with butter or margarine and artificially
sweetened fruit preserves
Half grapefruit, half cantaloupe, or any kind
of permitted fruit
Decaffeinated coffee

Mid-morning snack

Glass of milk and 2 or 3 saltines

Lunch

Cottage cheese salad with avocado or
unsweetened pineapple

Ham, ground steak, fish, or fowl
One cooked vegetable
One slice of protein bread (toasted if desired)
with butter or margarine

Mid-afternoon snack

Salted nuts

Dinner

Tossed green salad with or without small amount of
French or mayonnaise dressing
Roast beef or steak, latter preferably broiled
One cooked vegetable
Dietetic ice cream
Decaffeinated coffee

Bedtime snack

Glass of milk with thin slice of protein bread or
dietetic peanut butter and 2 or 3 saltines

THINGS TO REMEMBER ABOUT YOUR DIET

Milk

Children up to 12 years old need at least a pint of milk
daily, and adolescents need at least 1½ pints of milk
daily. Adults generally need a pint of milk daily, but
there are some adults who do not need and cannot
digest that much. If other mineral products are
served, the amount of milk may be reduced: 1½
ounces of regular cheese or 2 or 3 scoops of dietetic
(sugarless) ice cream count as a cup of milk. Raw,

pasteurized, canned, or powdered milk all have about the same food value.

Water

Drink lots of water. I suggest you drink the equivalent of 6 or 8 glasses of water (1½ to 2 quarts) daily. Other fluids—such as decaffeinated coffee, milk, or fruit juice—may be counted in the amount of liquid suggested above. I have read that a person who takes digitalis or has a poorly compensated heart disease should not drink much water, that six or eight glasses of water might throw him into more acute decompensation, and that for such a person one glass of water a day is probably safe.

Vitamins

Vitamins (whether taken in foods or as vitamin supplements) are foods, not medicines. Vitamins A and D, if taken in excess, can be toxic and frequently cause insomnia, headaches, restlessness, and irritability. Unless taken over a prolonged length of time and in exorbitant amounts, the toxic condition caused by excessive vitamin supplements generally disappears after use is discontinued. Remember, we get vitamin D from the sun, and some of our foods are enriched and fortified with additional vitamins. Taking excessive amounts of citrus fruits and their juices and ascorbic acid (vitamin C) supplements over a long period of time may produce an alkalized system, indicated by nasal itching and sometimes by small fissures in the nose, as well as by headaches, restlessness, and inability to sleep. This condition may be corrected by temporarily discontinuing the use of ascorbic acid foods and vitamin C supplements, and by the temporary administration of hydrochloric acid by your doctor.

Meats, Fish, and Poultry

One can, of course, overdo anything, but on this diet you are expected to eat meats, fish and poultry. I recommend that you eat liver frequently. You should eat eggs at least three times a week. If your physician has you on a low cholesterol diet, you must follow his recommendations about all cholesterol foods, including eggs, and disregard anything stated here to the contrary.

Mid-meal and Bedtime Snacks

Keep in mind always that your purpose in eating these snacks is to keep your blood sugar level as stable as possible. You are not to have six or seven meals a day, only three, and your regular meals are to be smaller because of your snacks. I have eaten almost every kind of food at snack time. The ones I have enjoyed most are fresh fruits, salted nuts, cheeses, peanut butter, milk, dietetic ice cream, beans, dietetic candies, and bits of fresh vegetables. At first you may be inclined to overdo on the snacks, but you will soon learn the proper amounts you should eat. After you have been on the diet a month or so, you may find you do not need to snack and that your three daily meals supply all the foods you need.

If you think of your diet as the beginning of a wonderful new experience in the field of nutrition and health, rather than a boring something to be tolerated for a year or so, I am sure you will find it rewarding and enjoyable. It was part of the gateway to a new life for me, and I hope you will find it as fascinating and profitable as I did.

Plan your meals and then enjoy them. Meal patterns vary in various parts of the United States and at various seasons of the year. Before 1959, I ate meals from a sense of duty—generally eating too fast and paying either little or no attention to what I ate, mostly wondering whether I was eating foods to which I was allergic. Now, I like to take an hour or more to eat a seafood dinner or an Oklahoma steak, and find as much pleasure in so doing as I do when I see two of the nation's leading college football teams play or when I sit in the grandstand watching a close major league baseball game.

7.

VITAMINS AND ENZYMES

MUCH HAS BEEN written about the body's daily vitamin requirements. Most physicians take the view that a well balanced diet contains most, if not all, of the essential vitamins. Nearly all doctors are of the opinion that there are times when certain vitamin supplements should be prescribed for some patients. Taking vitamins indiscriminately for any and all diseases, however, is looked upon with disfavor by the medical profession.

I am not inclined to start an argument with my medical friends about vitamins, but I believe their assumption that a well balanced diet furnishes all of the needed vitamins overlooks one question: "How many people have a well balanced diet daily?" What I know about the most common eating habits and what I have learned from my studies in nutrition have convinced me that few people have a well balanced diet.

Just as money is wasted on some unnecessary vitamin supplements, so is it wasted on erroneously prescribed medicines. Nevertheless, it would be ridiculous for me to say that I am not going to call a doctor when I become ill because my hypoglycemic condition was not correctly diagnosed until 1959. There is no doubt in my mind that for the remainder of my life I will take some vitamin A, B, C, D, and E supplements whenever I feel that I need them.

In my opinion, some vitamins are more closely related to allergies than others. I have already talked about pantothenic acid, and I want to tell you about my experiences with vitamin E.

This vitamin has been one of the most controversial subjects in medicine in the United States. Most doctors contend that we get a sufficient amount of vitamin E in our normal diet, whereas other American doctors, certainly in the minority, take the view that many patients need to take supplements of vitamin E daily. There have been reports of improvement and cure of diseases of the cardiovascular system from the addition of vitamin E to the diet. Other doctors have scoffed at such claims as being fantastic and unreasonable and have asserted that vitamin E could not have played such a role.

Doctors in Canada and Europe generally have a more positive attitude to the use of vitamin E supplements in treating specific diseases than have American physicians. I accidentally came across some Canadian medical publications which stated, in substance, that vitamin E plays an important role physiologically in inhibiting or reducing the tendency of oxygen to combine with other substances and produce a toxic condition. Stated another way, they asserted that with many people oxygen combines with other elements to form toxic compounds and that vitamin

E is an antioxidant. One article stated that because of this reduction-oxidation property, vitamin E is important in the end stages of carbohydrate metabolism.

These articles intrigued me for several reasons. I asked myself these questions: (1) Is it possible that a lack of vitamin E caused me to have breathing difficulties? (2) Were the nasal (rhinitis) attacks which followed the eating of certain foods at least partially caused by a toxic compound resulting from oxygen combining with some substance or substances in the offending food? (3) In the case that the answer to question 2 is Yes, would vitamin E supplement inhibit the formation of the toxic compound? (4) Was it possible that the "oxygen-combining" theory of these Canadian physicians was more correct than the "allergen sensitivity" theory of most American doctors?

The only way I knew to get the answers to these questions was to experiment with vitamin E. In 1956, I secured a large bottle of wheat germ capsules, the most potent I could find, and began taking several each day. All sorts of difficulties followed. I didn't sleep well at night; I was more nervous than usual during the daytime and my allergies worsened. I had a dull headache all of the time I was taking the wheat germ oil. After a few weeks of agony, I gave up my vitamin E experiment, threw away the remainder of the wheat germ capsules, and decided anyone who tried to be his own doctor surely had a fool for a patient.

Early in 1960, while I was making remarkable progress with the antihypoglycemia diet and adrenal cortex injections, I came across another medical article about vitamin

E. My first inclination was not to read it. I was certain I had read enough medical quackery about vitamin E to last a lifetime. Curiosity was too much for me, however, so I read the article. It stated that a patient going on vitamin E supplement should not take more than 100 units a day for the first week or ten days, since the vitamin has a tendency to raise the blood pressure and cause some of the symptoms I experienced from taking 1,000 or more units. It was further reported that patients who are allergic to wheat germ oil can sometimes tolerate natural dry vitamin E, made from wheat, soybeans, and other vegetable products.

For nearly a month, I weighed the pros and cons of trying vitamin E supplement again. One day I bought 100 capsules of dry vitamin E complex made from natural vegetable products. I took one capsule each day for 14 days and nothing of importance happened. I then started taking six capsules, 600 units, daily. After a week, I noticed my breathing was easier. I continued taking 600 units of vitamin E daily for several months until I discontinued taking the capsules for a few days because the vitamin had been stored in my body in sufficient quantity and I was getting some toxic effects from it. I was not sleeping as well as usual and was a little restless. I resumed taking one capsule daily, and since then, I have found this amount sufficient.

The effect of the vitamin was phenomenal. Instead of using only the upper part of my lungs to breathe, I seemed to be using all parts of my lungs in breathing. The nasal passages opened as they did when I took astringent nasal drops, and my hearing improved as my nose and throat cleared up. Whether my ability to eat foods to which I had been allergic was due to my new diet, the adrenal cortex shots, or the vitamin E supplement, I do not know, but I believe that all three had some part in it.

I know of no other allergic person who has benefited from vitamin E. As far as I know, the physicians who have had such wonderful success in helping allergics with the antihypoglycemia diet and the adrenal cortex extract injections have not used vitamin E supplements extensively.

Many physicians believe there may be some relationship between vitamin C and the production of the adrenal cortex hormones, in view of the high concentration of this vitamin in the adrenals. It is interesting to note that all commercial oral adrenal cortex extract tablets offered for sale, as far as I have been able to discover, are fortified with vitamin C.

The vitamins physicians most often prescribe in cases of adrenal cortex deficiency are pyridoxine (vitamin B_6) and vitamin B_{12}. In view of my experiences with vitamins, it seems to me that vitamin E and pantothenic acid might well be added in some cases.

Enzymology is another branch of biochemistry, or the chemistry of life, about which even the experts have much to learn. Fifty years ago, enzymology was in its infancy as a branch of nutritional science concerned with the digestion of foods. It has grown in medical importance through the years, and we may now be on the threshold of discoveries that will give all of us a richer and fuller

life and even provide the means for conquering and preventing most of the now-considered incurable diseases.

Is all of this just a wild figment of my imagination? I
don't think so. On September 19, 1961, in an article in
The New York Times, Dr. Ines Mandel of Columbia University reported to the American Chemical Society that
he, in association with Betty B. Cohen, had discovered a
bacterium that produces elastase, an enzyme, which,
coated with a substance called elastin, is thought to control the elasticity of the artery walls. You and I may live
to see the day when medical science will be able to prevent hardening of the arteries. Others may live to see
other miraculous discoveries in biochemistry when scientists will have learned nature's secrets sufficiently to stop
arteriosclerosis.

On April 27, 1962, *The New York Times* stated that
Canadian physicians reporting to the American Academy
of Neurology cited evidence that the brains of persons
afflicted with Parkinson's disease showed abnormally low
concentrations of two related chemicals called dopamine
and serotonin. They speculated that a deficiency of an
enzyme called dopadecarboxylase might be at least partly
responsible for these deficiencies. The article went on to
say that these doctors attempted to correct this lack of
enzymes by giving patients doses of the compounds from
which the body normally makes dopamine. Results were
described as impressive but temporary. Here, at last, is a
ray of hope for the more than one million Americans suffering from the presently incurable Parkinson's disease.

Thousands upon thousands of people suffering from

thrombophlebitis have been saved from death by enzymatic miracles. Yet it was only on June 27, 1954, that *The American Weekly* reported the story of how John Allen, after having arranged his own funeral, was able to leave the hospital in a month and lead a normal life after Dr. Irving Innerfield, an eminent enzymologist at New York's Mount Sinai Hospital, was called into the case. The article stated that Dr. Innerfield injected tryspin into one of Allen's muscles. Dr. Innerfield was quoted as having said that tryspin dissolves protein and that the injection of this catalyst starts a series of chemical reactions which thin out blood and allow it to flow freely through the veins.

Enzymes control all of our body functions. We know much about vitamins and their importance to our health because vitamins have been glamorized by pharmaceutical-manufacturing companies for years. We know little about the 700 known enzymes without which vitamins would be worthless. In fact, many of the vitamins are coenzymes. As the *Columbus Health Bulletin* said in 1961: "They [enzymes] control man as they control all life, from the instant of conception to the moment he dies, his successes and failures, his characteristics and personality, his complete destiny."

On July 12, 1962, an article appearing in the *Flint Journal* (Michigan) reported that doctors have learned that schizophrenic patients secrete 58 per cent less enzyme cholinesterase than do normal persons. Perhaps enzymologists, working with psychiatrists, will at some future time be able to help us maintain mental health just as doctors are now able to fortify us against polio. That doesn't seem too unreasonable.

You and I should be thankful that we live in the fabulous age of the study of enzymes. Scientists have barely entered this wonderful fairyland. What they will discover about these catalysts (substances having the power to cause other substances to produce chemical changes in living things) only time can tell. I hope I am among the living when many more of these secrets are revealed.

8.

YOU NEED THE MINERALS TOO

THE BODY NEEDS about 13 different minerals, all of which must be obtained from the antihypoglycemia diet. The three minerals most likely to be present in our bodies in insufficient amounts are calcium, iron, and iodine. Ninety per cent of the body's ash consists of calcium and phosphorus. Ninety-nine per cent of the calcium and 80 per cent of the phosphorus are found in the skeletal tissues and teeth. None of the other required minerals even approaches one per cent of the total body composition.

Calcium

Absorption of dietary calcium takes place in the small intestine. Normal gastric hydrochloric acid and the presence of vitamin D in the system facilitate the process.

Oxalic acid has an adverse effect on the absorption of calcium, although the amounts of dietary calcium lost ordinarily through calcium oxalate formation are not serious. Because of their oxalic content, large quantities of rhubarb and spinach may interfere with efficient calcium absorption.

Phytic acid also has an adverse effect on calcium absorption. Because of their phytic acid content, large amounts of whole-wheat cereals may interfere with the efficient absorption of calcium. An excess of fats in the intestine reduces calcium absorption, whereas a small amount of fat improves the process.

The blood circulates the calcium absorbed from the food through the body; the parathyroid hormones regulate calcium blood levels. Calcium absorption is reversible, and calcium in the bones may be withdrawn to maintain normal blood levels during periods of calcium deprivation.

Normally, the kidneys excrete any excess of blood calcium over ten milligrams per 100 millimeters. Calcium is also excreted through the feces.

Among children, rickets is the principal calcium deficiency disease. Among adults, a calcium, phosphorus, vitamin D deficiency is called osteomalacia, characterized by softening of the bones.

Milk and dairy products, shellfish, egg yolk, soybeans and green vegetables are good sources of calcium. In America, our best sources of this mineral are milk, cheese, and bone meal.

Phosphorus

This mineral has more body functions than any other. With calcium, it lends rigidity to the bones and teeth. About 80 per cent of the body's phosphorus is found in the skeletal tissue and teeth and the other 20 per cent is located in the body fluids and in every cell. Phosphorus metabolism is important in muscle-energy and nerve-tissue metabolism, in carbohydrate, protein, and fat metabolism, in normal blood chemistry, in skeletal growth and tooth development, as well as in the transport of fatty acids. It is also a component of many enzyme systems.

About 70 per cent of the phosphorus ingested is absorbed in the body. Vitamin D and a normal acid medium assist phosphorus absorption. The common foods which meet calcium and protein needs are usually simultaneously able to supply the required phosphorus.

The protein-rich foods—meat, fish, eggs and poultry—are excellent sources of this mineral. Milk, cheese, nuts and the legumes are also good sources of phosphorus.

Iron

This mineral plays an essential role in oxygen transport by the blood and in cellular respiration. It constitutes only .004 per cent of the body (4.5 grams in an average adult). Approximately one gram of this iron is stored in the liver and spleen.

Iron deficiency in man is one form of anemia, which may develop from inadequate diet or poor absorption. Blood loss, particularly chronic blood loss, may lead to anemia. Persons who harbor intestinal parasites or who suffer from bleeding hemorrhoids, bleeding ulcers, or recurrent nose bleeds are prone to iron deficiency.

The Food and Nutrition Board of the National Research Council recommends a daily intake of 10 to 15 milligrams of iron for adults and adolescents, and from 7 to 12 milligrams daily for children. These foods, in decreasing order of excellence, are good sources of iron: liver, heart, kidney, liver sausage, lean meats, shellfish, egg yolk, dried beans and other legumes, dried fruits, nuts, green leafy vegetables, whole grain and enriched cereals, and molasses. That milk is a poor source of iron accounts for the fact that infants must have foods containing iron to supplement milk.

Copper

The human diet usually supplies an adequate amount of copper. The daily minimum requirement of two milligrams of copper is supplied by even a poor diet. Copper is stored in the liver. Milk is low in copper, but a newborn baby has a stored-up liver supply of copper five to ten times greater than the supply of this mineral stored in an adult's liver. The best sources of copper are oysters, liver, beef, nuts, and mushrooms.

Iodine

This mineral is an essential nutrient since it plays such an important part in the formation of thyroid hormones, which regulate the metabolic rate. The output of the thyroid gland is affected by the availability of iodine. If the iodine supply is inadequate, the gland increases its secretory activity and enlarges until it becomes a goiter.

Iodine is absorbed from the small intestine. It is found in the blood as both inorganic iodine and protein-bound iodine. Optimal requirements for iodine in the adult range from .15 to .30 milligrams per day.

Foods grown on iodine-poor soil contain insufficient iodine for meeting human needs. Goiter is frequently prevalent in those regions where there is a deficiency of iodine in the soil. They are sometimes called "goiter belts" or "goiter regions."

Among natural foods, the best sources of iodine are sea foods and vegetables grown on iodine-rich land, or kelp. The major source of iodine in America is iodized salt.

Cobalt

This mineral is known to compose about 4 per cent of vitamin B_{12}. It has been theorized that cobalt, being so closely associated with vitamin B_{12}, may assist in preventing anemia. Cobalt is found in most foods and there is no known human requirement of the mineral. It has been speculated that cobalt may play a part in the normal metabolism of human growth.

Zinc, Manganese, Molybdenum, and Magnesium

A normal diet supplies these minerals although we do not know what minimum requirement is. A true dietary deficiency of magnesium has not been found, but there are cases on record of severe illnesses and chronic alcoholism where there was a prolonged administration of a diet free from magnesium; the subjects had muscular tremor, uncoordinated movements, and, sometimes, convulsions. These persons readily responded to the administration of magnesium.

Fluorine

This mineral is important since it is normally present in bones and teeth to prevent dental caries. Although it is found in many foods, we acquire most of our fluorine from drinking water. The average daily diet, including foods cooked in water, provides .25 to .32 milligrams of fluoride. During the period of tooth formation, the child's diet should contain an additional supplement of fluoride equal to about 1 mg. daily. Many dentists have applied a 2 per cent sodium fluoride solution directly to the teeth, especially of younger people, and have reported that it was effective in controlling dental caries.

Many cities and communities now add sodium fluoride to their water supplies in an effort to prevent dental caries among the young. Fluoridated water usually contains 1 ppm of fluorine. (It is claimed that water containing as much as 1.8 ppm of fluorine may produce mottling of the dental enamel.)

Sodium and Potassium

About .2 per cent of the body is sodium, most of which is found in the body fluids. Under normal conditions, 90 per cent of ingested sodium is excreted in the urine, either as sodium chloride or sodium phosphate. Under conditions of intense perspiration, sweat may become the main vehicle of excretion. Prolonged perspiration may lead to a sodium depletion, accompanied by muscular cramps, weakness, and headache. Some occupations require increased salt intake to replace loss of sodium chloride. Where there is an adrenal cortical deficiency, an additional intake of salt is recommended.

The normal daily salt requirement ranges from 2 to 20 grams, more salt being required in proportion to the amount of water taken. After recurrent vomiting or protracted diarrhea, a special need for sodium chloride, as well as for potassium, arises.

Potassium is present in a lesser degree in the body than is sodium, and is mostly found in the cells. The muscles contain about six times as much potassium as sodium. Potassium has a close connection with muscle function, as well as heart function, and, along with calcium, it helps maintain nerve irritability or excitability; potassium also plays a part in carbohydrate metabolism. Dietary potassium deficiency does not exist under ordinary circumstances. Potassium deficiency results from some diseases—not necessarily chronic—and is manifested in muscular weakness, nervous irritability, cardiac irregularities, and sometimes, mental confusion. Excessive concentrations of potassium, usually caused by kidney disease or dehydration, may result in a serious cardiac condition if not corrected. The dietary need for potassium is roughly the same as that for sodium.

Water

This mineral is second only to oxygen in maintaining life. Water is not only an essential nutrient, but the major component of the body as well. It is the body's vehicle for chemical transport and the medium in which practically all metabolic reactions involving other nutrients take place. The Food and Nutrition Board recommends, under conditions of moderate temperature and normal exercise, an intake of one milliliter of water for each calorie of food.

Other mineral elements

Sulfur, aluminum, silicon, and bromide, while always present in the body, have not as yet been demonstrated to affect normal metabolism. Investigators may later show that these elements (although present in small quantities) as well as some others, such as arsenic, nickel, boron, and selenium, play roles in metabolism, digestion, and mental processes not even contemplated at this time.

9.

ALCOHOL AND
THE ADRENAL GLANDS

DR. TINTERA, WHO was a charter member of the New York Medical Committee on Alcoholism, and is an authority on the endocrine treatment of alcoholics, states in one of his published medical papers: "Show me an alcoholic, any alcoholic, and I will show you adrenal glands exhausted by alcohol."

Most of us have grown accustomed to thinking of the chronic alcoholics, who probably include five or six million Americans, as suffering from a disease, *alcoholism*. We haven't given much thought to how alcoholism should or could be treated, and we have generally assumed that alcoholism must have been caused by some early emotional trauma and that it is the problem of the alcoholic and his psychiatrist, or of Alcoholic Anonymous, to get the alcoholic back on the right track.

The endocrinologists who hold that alcoholism is not a disease in itself, but a symptom of a functional disturbance in the cortex of the adrenal glands, with the same mental abberations sometimes found in hypoglycemic states, have found that alcoholism responds well to the endocrine therapy.

Dr. Tintera, in a paper published in the *New York Journal of Medicine* on December 15, 1956, reported that he had successfully treated more than 200 alcoholics, many of whom had been members of Alcoholics Anonymous for several years. Dr. Tintera proceeded in those cases on the assumption that alcoholism, like hay fever, asthma, migraine, or hives, is a symptom of a glandular disorder. He does not discount the value of the wonderful work done by the Alcoholics Anonymous organization.

I have read every book I have been able to find relating to the work of Alcoholics Anonymous. Without going into detail as to how A.A. works or for what it stands, I know it has done more for mankind during the past 30 years than has any other similarly organized group in the history of the world during the same period of time.

Alcoholics call upon general practitioners to treat them for heart disease and cancer (in that order of frequency) more than for alcoholism. Doctors tell us, however, that alcoholism is growing and that unless the present trend is reversed, alcoholism may become one of the most common diseases with which the general practitioners or family doctors will have to cope.

Now that we know more about alcoholism, the social stigma has been partially removed from alcoholism, and some hospitals admit alcoholics as patients. Due to the crowded conditions prevailing in most hospitals, these patients are kept for only a limited time. I am told that in some of our larger cities hospital facilities for treating alcoholics as alcoholics, and not as merely physically ill persons, have been established. In many states however, there are no hospitals or adequate facilities available for the treatment of these people, particularly if they are without funds to pay for such care.

Throughout the country, we have many farms or "alcoholic sanitaria," privately run by lay management (usually alcoholics themselves), where the "patients," or whatever they are called, are mistreated and misguided; and when whatever funds the alcoholic or his family has are gone, he returns to society worse off—if any change has occurred—than when he entered.

I think all physicians who have made an extensive study of alcoholism generally agree that the successful treatment of alcoholism requires the recognition that it has rightfully been placed in the classification of a psychosomatic disorder. However, physicians are not completely in agreement as to the part, if any, drug therapy, should and can play. This much can be said: those who contend that alcoholism is purely a psychic phenomenon are unable to show any appreciable percentage of recoveries through psychiatry alone. Those who contend that alcoholism is not primarily a psychic disorder, but rather an organic disease referable to the men of internal medicine, are unable to show any better record of recoveries than are the psychiatrists.

Dr. Tintera says that endocrinology is a requisite for the consummate treatment of the disorder. He points out that it is a well-known fact that the last person to recognize an alcoholic problem is the alcoholic himself.

Without considering those patients brought, intoxicated,

to the doctor by family pressure or a clash with the law, those who only desire to be sobered up, or those who come to the physician solely for help in getting over a hangover (without any intent of giving up drinking), Dr. Tintera goes into a discussion of those individuals who recognize they have an alcoholic problem and plead for help in getting over their craving for alcohol. He it talking about the patient who, after a long period of sobriety, wants to obtain permanent sobriety.

Dr. Tintera states that the recovered alcoholic consults his doctor because he is dissatisfied with his way of life, even if he has maintained sobriety for years. His symptoms are an aggravation of those that initiated his drinking.

Even when they have remained "dry," as A.A. puts it, for years, alcoholics usually have insatiable desires for sweets or carbohydrates in some form. They are frequently introverted and anti-social; they are dependent individuals who must regain their confidence and a desire to be productive and useful. Unless the patient is willing to give up drinking completely, he is wasting his time and that of the doctor. Even if he believes he can limit his drinking to a weekend cocktail, the treatment will be a complete failure. Until such time as the patient has conceded that total and complete alcoholic restriction from then on is necessary, failure of treatment is inevitable.

The tests the doctor gives are more detailed than those discussed in prior chapters, since the physician must determine—either at the start of the treatment or later—the amount of liver damage, if any, caused by the prolonged drinking. He also carefully checks to see if there has been any damage to the patient's kidneys. Upon completion of a thorough physical examination and complete history, three laboratory tests are routinely given: (1) urinalysis, (2) complete blood count, and (3) a glucose tolerance test. If the patient is found to be suffering from hypoadrenocorticism, he is put on the anti-hypoglycemia diet previously outlined, with one exception: it is a high protein, low carbohydrate, high fat diet, instead of the medium fat diet prescribed for non-alcoholic patients.

The patient is then given the adrenal cortex extract injections. As in other cases of hypoadrenocorticism, the length of the intervals between injections increases as the patient approaches the time when the injections may be discontinued.

Dr. Tintera believes that regular consultations of a psychiatric nature between the physician (generally a general practitioner or family doctor) and the patient, must continue indefinitely. The patient must be continually reassured by his doctor as he redirects him to a more fruitful outlook on life. There must be a rational medical explanation in layman's language of the emotional, psychological, hormonal ramifications of the patient's illness. When the patient is able to control and understand the hypoglycemic episodes discussed in prior chapters, he will be relieved of much of his tension.

It is a procedure that requires understanding and patience on the part of the physician, for he may expect some reverses as the treatment proceeds. Many times the patient, without returning to liquor, will indicate that he can't go through with the treatment; and there will be times when the patient is very depressed and needs more than usual reassurance. As the treatment progresses, the patient's entire outlook will improve; there will be a lessening of his negativism and a reversal of the personality traits present at the beginning of the treatment.

Within the first few months of treatment, endocrine balance is well established. As the patient regains physiological, endocrinological, and mental balance, he becomes aware of his social obligations and loses his compulsions, apprehensions, and inhibitions. We then have a clear-thinking, calm, outgoing, and energetic individual.

The patient must be taught that if he allows his blood sugar to reach hypoglycemic levels again, many of his original emotional problems will return—along with a craving for carbohydrates, more specifically, alcohol.

Pyridoxine (vitamin B6) is frequently given as a valuable adjunct in rehabilitating alcoholics. Although alcoholism has never been one of my problems, a dermatologist once prescribed vitamin B6 supplement for a scaly, itching dermatitis which had been annoying me a long time. This vitamin supplement soon cured my skin condition. The only reason for mentioning this is that I have noticed that a number of alcoholics brought before me as a district judge on various charges had noticeable skin diseases on their faces, particularly around their eyes and ears.

Alcohol is the adrenals' number-one enemy. Someone born with strong adrenals will probably be able to drink heavily for a long time before he becomes an alcoholic. The chances are he can drink in moderation all of his life without alcohol injuring him seriously. If an individual was born with weak adrenals, or if his adrenals have been damaged by disease, he will not be able to drink very long until alcohol does him lasting damage.

We speculate why one man can drink heavily for years and not become an alcoholic, while another becomes an alcoholic after drinking a few years. To say that a person will become an alcoholic if he is a heavy drinker for a certain number of years is as absurd as to say a man will develop heart disease when his weight reaches a certain number of pounds over what it should be.

Body chemistry has no use for alcohol; its whole aim is to get rid of it. To do so, it must convert alcohol into carbon dioxide and water. This chemical conversion takes place largely in the liver and it continues as long as there is any alcohol in the body. The adrenal cores secrete their stress hormones; the whole system of endocrine glands is roused, and the adrenal casing hormones direct glucose into the blood from the liver, where the glucose has been stored as glycogen.

Blood sugar level goes up, so the islets of the pancreas pour insulin into the blood to lower it. One drink will keep this chemical chaos going for a few hours. If you drink no more than that you feel quite normal again after a brief letdown. The whiplashing the adrenals receive is not long and not severe, so the glands can recover quickly.

If you have a lot of drinks you wind up with more or less exhausted adrenals and with what we call a hangover—a low blood sugar condition. You feel terrible, listless, tired and depressed, have a headache, and are unable to think clearly. If you don't drink again your adrenals will recover in a day or a week (depending on the strength of your glands), and you will feel normal again.

But, for the man or woman who becomes an alcoholic things don't work out that way. While the adrenals are still more or less exhausted, and while the blood sugar level is down, the individual starts drinking again in order to feel better; the same chemical process begins, and, unless he stops drinking, the person finally collapses. This is the chemical merry-go-round to which an alcoholic is chained.

As glycogen is taken from the liver without being replaced through proper nutrition, more fat collects in the liver. The alcoholic gets his calories from alcohol, and these calories are quickly metabolized. The inevitable result, unless drinking is at least temporarily stopped, is general physical collapse and probable death caused by a ruined liver and pancreas.

The physical basis of alcoholism is, then, a functional disturbance of the adrenals and a real, organic need for sugar. If that were all there is to alcoholism, it would be one of the easiest diseases of all to curb. All the doctor would need to do would be to put the alcoholic on a diet that places little strain on the adrenals and administer adrenal cortex extract until the adrenals rehabilitated themselves.

However, alcoholism is not that simple a disease. It involves the whole person, the body, the mind, and the emotions. After the alcoholic's physical craving for liquor is gone, treatment must continue until such time as the person's mental and emotional difficulties are under control. Dr. Tintera has observed that an alcoholic, *any alcoholic,* can be sobered permanently if he has a strong enough will to stop drinking completely and forever. That doesn't mean he will have to continue with the adrenal cortex extract, but it does mean he may have to remain on the diet for an indefinite length of time.

I am sure you have known alcoholics who have stopped drinking and have substituted sugar or sugar products for alcohol. The physical craving for alcohol will continue as long as the alcoholic keeps his chemical merry-go-round in motion, whether from alcohol or other quickly-absorbed carbohydrates, such as sugar, candies, pastries, sweetened soft drinks, cakes, pies, cereals, potatoes, corn, dates, raisins, honey, and spaghetti. The adrenals and the islets of the pancreas will carry on their tug of war over lowering and raising the blood sugar level, and the alcoholic, although "dry," will feel miserable most of the time.

The view that alcoholism is a complicated disease, and not evidence of a depraved mind, is held by a minority— but certainly an enlightened minority—of our people. When we try to determine why any alcoholic started to drink, we have a difficult question to answer. When we ask why he continued to drink more and more as time went on, we have a more difficult question to answer. In trying to get the answers to some of these questions, I have talked with many alcoholics who have appeared in my courts.

Since my attitude toward these people has always been one of sympathy and not of condemnation, practically all of them have given me truthful answers, *as far as they*

knew, even when I, as a trial judge, imposed penitentiary
sentences for offenses they had committed. They could
not explain their early problems, if any, because of my
lack of psychiatric training and the lack of time for more
than casual interviews.

I was astounded at the effects intoxication had on them.
Alcohol, so they said, gave them a sense of importance,
relieved their apprehensions and anxieties, and gave them
a temporary feeling of well-being, a reversal of their usual
feelings of inferiority. Some of them told me they thought
they got drunk to punish themselves for something—they
did not know what. I did not have to remind any of them
that what they told me were rationalizations; they admitted that as a part of their answers. More than half of
them said, in substance: "I know I am running from something; I don't know what it is." We can call these people
cowards, but aren't we all cowards in some way or another?

Medical science is doing a wonderful work in helping
alcoholics rehabilitate. I think some doctors' initial approach is wrong. They tell an alcoholic that some day he
will be able, or *perhaps* be able, to drink again. Their
excuse for doing so is that they want to give the alcoholic
something to "hang on to"; otherwise they fear, he will
never try to help himself.

I think a doctor should never lie to a patient unless it
is necessary to save the patient's life or prevent immediate
serious injury. If, in the back of his mind, the alcoholic
believes he will be able to drink again, he is liable to

cheat and believe he can fool his doctor by taking a drink or a few drinks without the doctor's knowledge.

Until an alcoholic knows that he has a drinking problem and that he may have it the rest of his life, and until he has absolutely and completely determined, without any reservation, to give up drinking forever, *he is beyond the help of medical science.* Doctors by the dozens have agreed with me on the statement I have just made. They have further agreed with me on these things:

1. The alcoholic must be made to understand that one drink anytime and any place will again enslave him.

2. He must be told that every hour and every day he abstains he will more and more appreciate and enjoy the concrete benefits of a properly functioning glandular system; that people and the world will look better to him every day he goes without liquor. The temptation to take just a little drink is greatest at a time of stress or grief, and that is the most dangerous time. If the alcoholic gets by such a period without a drink, he wins a great victory.

3. There is no such a person as a "cured" or "recovered" alcoholic. The patient should be told that it will be impossible for him to always run from alcohol and that the best answer for him to give when would-be friends insist that he drink, is to tell them he is an alcoholic and can never drink again; then, he must stick to it.

4. The physician should, in sympathetic and understandable language, explain to the patient the treatment and the reasons for the treatment.

5. Psychotherapy by the doctor is more important than medication and diet. While the physician must at all times

have a sympathetic and understanding attitude, more
help will come to the patient if he is the one who initiates
the inquiries and attempts to answer his own questions.
The alcoholic is usually a sensitive person who resents any
lecturing or sermonizing by his doctor or by members of
his family.

6. Sometimes the husband or wife of an alcoholic needs
counselling by the doctor; the spouse's attitude might have
to be changed so that he or she will be able to assist in
educating and directing the alcoholic to a new life of
happiness, usefulness, and productivity.

Unless the physician likes people and has a sincere
desire to help them, he will not be interested in trying to
help an alcoholic rehabilitate himself. Every alcoholic
who comes to a doctor with a sincere desire to be rehabilitated and a willingness to conform to whatever is
required of him, presents a challenge to the doctor as
great, if not greater, than the challenge which an unusual,
delicate, and difficult operation presents to a great surgeon. If I had my life to live over I would study medicine
instead of law so that I might be able to try to help do
some of the things I have talked about in this chapter.

Doctors have observed that they never knew a diabetic
who became an alcoholic. There are alcoholics, however,
who have become diabetics. These people burdened their
livers and pancreatic glands to such an extent that both
became diseased, and the islands of Langerhans, that part
of the pancreas that manufactures insulin, became unable
to furnish normal daily amounts of insulin.

A well-known eastern physician wrote me: "I would

not for a moment discount the wonderful work of Alcoholics Anonymous. They have dried up more men and women than have all of the doctors in America combined. However, every medical adviser to Alcoholics Anonymous I ever knew believed that the best way to rehabilitate alcoholics was by the glandular treatment and psychotherapy."

The cost to the nation caused by the excessive use of alcohol is now estimated to be in the neighborhood of a billion dollars annually. This is only a part of the overall cost. The thousands upon thousands of divorce cases that have gone through my courts have provided me with first-hand information about the tragedies, the suffering, and the ruined lives of those who never drank but were the victims of alcoholism as much as, if not more than, the alcoholics themselves.

There is no escaping the responsibility we all have for the high rate of alcoholism in this nation. We must recognize the social anomaly that makes social drinking respectable and leads a weak and dependent character into alcoholism. We salve our consciences by saying, "it's a free country," the one who will later become an alcoholic, "doesn't have to drink unless he wants to do so," and, after all, "it's really none of our business who drinks or how much he drinks."

After we have furnished the opportunity and encouraged a weak and dependent individual to become an alcoholic, we become rather high and mighty in our attitude toward him. "He's gotten himself in that condition; let him get out of it." It's not difficult for us to become self-righteous about our social drinking. Sometimes we become big-hearted in our willingness to help our former drinking friends. If they don't have any money to get help for themselves, which we know is often the case, we don't grumble too much about paying our share of taxes for public institutions to help the destitute alcoholics. I am sure that our hypocrisy about our responsibility for some of the results of social drinking is at least partially responsible for the callous manner in which we treat most alcoholics.

Doctors tell us alcohol is not addicting, like morphine and cocaine, but it is definitely habit-forming. It is dangerous because it is connected with a ritual, such as communal drinking, which has social approbation. Why then does the alcoholic apparently have such an uncontrollable appetite for liquor? If the forces of psychological stimulation are the sole causes of irresistible craving for alcohol, how can we explain the hangover or the alcoholic's inability to keep from pouring liquor into his body when he knows that no pleasure, only suffering, can come to him?

Never having drunk much liquor, I can only base my conclusions on my own experiences. Similarly, under the established rules of evidence, a lay witness may state opinions in courts of law if he first states the facts upon which his opinions are based. Many, many times I have had as uncontrollable a desire for sugar as any alcoholic ever had for liquor. The more sugar I ate, the more sugar I wanted. Because I was sober, I knew better than the alcoholic what sugar would do to me.

No advocate of the theory that alcoholism is psychic

and psychic only will ever be able to convince me that my uncontrollable craving for sugar was all psychological. My body was crying out for food; although I was overweight, I was at least partially starving. When I ate sugar, the glucose that entered my bloodstream made me feel good.

Fortunately for me, I went for the sugar instead of the alcohol. I believe that I had as many emotional and mental problems to face when I reached maturity as does the average person who becomes an alcoholic. Yet, my problems were easier to solve than they would have been had I become an alcoholic, because sugar or other ordinary carbohydrate food does not damage the body, the brain, the mind, and the personality as alcohol does.

When I went on the antihypoglycemic diet and began taking the adrenal cortex injections, my problem was simple—regaining my health. Sugar had done no damage to me that could not be repaired easily and in a fairly short time.

At the beginning of any rehabilitation program, the alcoholic's problems are complex and difficult. His body chemistry was out of order to begin with, and by drinking he brought upon himself all the ills of alcoholism. He has a rough road ahead of him, even if every person he meets is kind, considerate, and sympathetic. Most of us are moralists when dealing with the other person's faults and weaknesses. We are far more charitable with our own faults and weaknesses than we are with those of our friends and relatives. The alcoholic frequently finds himself in a world where few are tolerant, sympathetic, or kind to him.

After he no longer has a physical need for liquor and has determined, with all the will power he possesses, never to take another drink, the alcoholic is, in some ways, like a little child learning to walk. He falters, he stumbles, he may even fall down; but every day he is more determined than ever to succeed in conquering his alcoholism. The most despicable character I can think of is one who deliberately does something to impede the alcoholic in his determination to "walk as he once did."

To my way of thinking, the secret of the success of Alcoholics Anonymous is its humanness; it gives the new member the feeling—perhaps for the first time in years—that he has friends who understand and appreciate what he is up against. It is a form of mass psychotherapy conducted by laymen who, by nature, are sympathetic to their fellow men.

A.A. was not organized to furnish medical treatment to its members; that they must get themselves. However, it has given the members of America's low and middle income classes the opportunity, that formerly only the rich could afford, to rebuild their lives. A.A. is a great success if for no other reason than that it is effective among the alcoholics who seek its aid.

10.

TRACKING DOWN
THE NUMBER ONE KILLER

EVERY PHYSICIAN WHO has successfully treated allergy cases with the antihypoglycemia diet and adrenal cortex extract injections has observed the improvement in the general health of his patients.

Doctors with whom I have corresponded have commented on how the diet and medication reduced the amount of cholesterol in the bloodstream. Physicians have been telling us for years that lowering cholesterol prevents and sometimes cures athcrosclerosis, a condition where blood passages are narrowed, with the result that clots adhere to the linings of the vessels, stopping the normal flow of blood to the heart. This causes what the doctors refer to as a "coronary occlusion," or, what the layman speaks of as a "heart attack."

When I began my research I was only interested in allergy cases; however, when both patients and doctors told me, in substance, that the diet and medication discussed in prior chapters seemed to prevent and hasten recovery from coronary attacks, I was intrigued. Because so many judges and lawyers have recently suffered heart attacks, I was anxious to know why a low carbohydrate, high protein diet and injections of the whole adrenal cortex extract might be beneficial in preventing attacks of the nation's "number one killer," coronary heart disease.

The answers given me by both doctors and laymen were convincing. They suggested that the clearing of fat and other sludge from the bloodstream was promoted by one or more of the following factors: (1) Eliminating pies, cakes, and other pastries from the diet, thus reducing the fat intake. (2) A diet rich in fruits and vegetables with a high vitamin C content, which, along with increased amounts of other vitamins, may be beneficial. (3) Eating apples, which are a good source of pectin, known to be an anti-cholesterol food element. (4) Attaining and maintaining normal weight while on the diet. (5) Reducing tensions and anxieties by means of diet and medication. (The effect is much the same as that of tranquilizing drugs —but without unfavorable side effects.)

A team of physicians in California, including Dr. Meyer Friedman and Dr. Ray H. Rosenman, both cardiologists, and Dr. Sanford O. Byers, a biochemist, have been working for years to determine the causes of coronary heart disease. These physicians had thousands of business executives as volunteers and made what was probably the most complete, massive study undertaken in the medical battle against coronary attacks.

Late in 1964, the Journal of the American Medical Association reported the findings of this medical team.

These physicians discovered that the administration of ACTH (adrenocorticotropin) to their volunteers after rich meals quickly cleared fat from the bloodstream. Tests made on these volunteers after they had been given the same rich food but not the ACTH showed that some of the fat remained in the bloodstream as long as 24 hours after the meals had been eaten.

Tests made by these California specialists on persons whose adrenal glands had been removed showed conclusively that ACTH by itself did not clear the bloodstream after rich meals.

As was observed in a prior chapter, ACTH stimulates the adrenals to produce more hormones. From the report of Drs. Friedman, Rosenman and Byers, we know that *malfunction of the adrenal glands is the basic cause of coronary heart disease*. These California doctors and many others are attempting to identify the adrenal hormone that apparently clears the bloodstream of excess fats and cholesterol. When this hormone is discovered, it will, without doubt, be produced synthetically and made available to physicians. Further testing will be necessary to determine whether the synthetic hormone can safely be used in coronary heart disease cases.

When Drs. Friedman and Rosenman made a report in 1958 to the American Heart Association that their tests had indicated that blood cholesterol level was not controlled solely by diet, they were greeted with dead silence.

It is axiomatic that if the adrenals are manufacturing all of their hormones in sufficient quantities, there is no necessity for stimulating them with ACTH.

How far medical researchers will go in proving that adequate hormone production by the adrenal glands prevents and, when induced, can cure a myriad of diseases, is as much the guess of one person as it is of another. It would appear that even now, with the medical knowledge of hypoglycemia and hypoadrenocorticism available to physicians, heart disease need not continue to be the nation's number one killer.

It seems to me that if we had a few large hypoglycemia foundations in America, it would not take long for physicians to be able to tell us the role, if any, that our adrenals play in our illnesses. Even before the eminent California doctors made their momentous discovery that some unknown hormone from the adrenal glands is responsible for removing fat, calcium, and other sludge from our bloodstreams, other physicians, sometimes family doctors, had become convinced that the adrenals had something to do with preventing and curing heart disease. These doctors did not have the time, the money, or the facilities to make the massive tests of the California physicians.

I have not attempted to summarize all of the findings and conclusions of Dr. Friedman and Dr. Rosenman. They found that aggressive, hard-driving men are subject to heart attack, and also that among men prone to coronary disease, high fat levels build up in the bloodstream. They have demonstrated that heart attacks can be fairly accurately predicted in men who showed no clinical evidence of coronary disease. Their report, in part, read: "The frequent heart attack after a heavy meal now becomes explicable to us."

I do not contend that the low carbohydrate, high protein diet and adrenal cortex extract medication constitute a "cure-all" for all diseases, but I am hopeful that in the next few years much medical research will be done to determine the role of the adrenal glands in all kinds of disease. I believe that if and when this is done, some of the reports will be as startling to both physicians and laymen as were the published results of the tests made by Dr. Friedman and Dr. Rosenman.

11.

A TREATMENT
THAT CURES ALLERGIES

WE WHO HAVE gotten over our allergies by a treatment so new that more than half of our practicing physicians readily admit they know little or nothing about it, owe a tremendous debt of gratitude to the medical pioneers in hypoglycemia and hypoadrenocorticism. They have not received the recognition they so justly deserve from the public or from the medical associations.

A letter from a professor at Massachusetts Institute of Technology is indicative of what is being done in all parts of the nation by physicians who have the courage, the knowledge, and the determination to restore health to our long-suffering hypoadrenocortics. The letter reads:

June 13, 1963

Dear Judge Blaine:

I am pleased to respond to your letter.

My eldest daughter Martha was essentially bedridden, had no appetite, suffered from insomnia, and was seriously underdeveloped for her age, which was then eight years. Her condition derived from chronic asthma, which had plagued her from approximately her first birthday and which had made impossible any of the physical activity normal for a young child; indeed, she missed over half of the first three years of school because of colds, flu, respiratory infections, and general sickliness. During this period, we continually consulted with the best allergy specialists available in Boston, submitting her to innumerable tests, treatments, and medications, all of which became progressively less effective. Compounding our difficulty was the fact that another child in our family of five daughters was exhibiting similar though less severe symptoms, as was my wife also; in many respects our home resembled a dispensary, with at least one, and usually several, persons ill and taking medicine against respiratory infection.

Using results of tests performed here at the Children's Medical Center and his supplementary personal observations, a physician diagnosed Martha's condition as extreme hypoadrenocorticism, thoroughly investigated our respective families' histories as related to and confirming her trouble, and commenced treatment of the child. Melodramatic though it may sound, the effects were immediately obvious. On the four-hour trip by auto to this doctor's office, she lay on an improvised bunk on the rear seat of the car with very little energy, appetite, or interest, and I carried her bodily, over my shoulder, from the parking lot into his office. Perhaps six hours later, when we were halfway home, she complained of hunger, walked unaided from the car to a roadside restaurant, ate a plateful of fried hamburgers and drank several glasses of milk, returned to the car unaided, and promptly fell asleep for the remainder of the journey.

Over the next several years, under this doctor's continued care and with the assistance of our local physician, Martha has continued to prosper; today she is robust, very athletic, rarely ill from any cause, does very well in her schoolwork, has an almost voracious appetite and could accurately be described as cured of asthma. The same can be said of her younger sister and of my wife; our entire family, by following the prescribed diet, now enjoys an unusually steady state of good health; and if any child needs to remain home from school for a day, or requires bed rest, it is something of an event—so much so that all of their teachers, with no prompting, have individually commented upon the unusual attendance records of all the children. To say we never become sick would be an exaggeration, but compared to our previous situation, the present one is a radical transformation for the better.

Perhaps because of my education and professional activities, I consistently evaluate a theory or an action by the results it produces and the effect it creates. The conventional treatments were not effective with my family; the care given produced the desired results in the three instances known to me intimately. Thus, I conclude that the analysis of the malfunction and treatment of it are correct. . . .

Another letter has come to me from a student with both a bachelor's degree and a master's degree, and who is now working toward his doctorate at Columbia University. The letter follows:

July 8, 1963

Dear Judge Blaine:

I have had an asthmatic condition all of my twenty-five years, having inherited same from my father. I can vividly recall how continually I suffered in my boyhood and adolescent days in Tennessee—not just for hours or a few days, but sometimes for as many as two consecutive weeks, particularly in the summer. Asthma powder and muscular injections of adrenalin provided my only intermittent relief. Otherwise, I was practically immobilized.

Somehow, I thought that all of this would end when I

moved to Buffalo, New York in 1951, at the age of 14. But it did not. I continued to have persistent wheezing and shortness of breath, along with severe attacks from time to time.

On occasion of one of the latter in 1955, I met an allergist; and this time, I not only thought that it all would end; I just knew that it would. Thus allergy tests and subsequent immunization treatments were begun in optimism, but the optimism proved to be only partially warranted. Yes, I was helped. The severe attacks became scattered to the point of having only about one a year for the last few years (1960-62). Only, the wheezing and shortness of breath continued as before, the difference being that I was able to control them better. But so doing required the continual use of a nebulizer and antihistamines. In fact, I do not recall a single day on which I did not use my nebulizer!

This was my state of health when I came to school in New York City in September, 1962. And unlike when I left Tennessee, I had no hope of a change this time; but, as fate would have it, change came anyway.

A physician began treating me in October, and change began immediately. On the very next day after I received my first treatment, I did not, for the first time since 1955, use my nebulizer or take an antihistamine. Also, within that first week, my shortness of breath became less pronounced. Even more, within a two-week period, I began to notice that I could read without getting as tired, that I could type without making as many errors, and that I could relax while writing. My condition, incidentally, had become such that my hand muscles would tighten when I wrote, or my hands would become very unsteady.

Today, ten months later, these changes persist. Wheezing and shortness of breath are things that I don't even think about any more. I work long hours (doing mental work) without becoming abnormally tired; I write without being nervous; and I type with greater accuracy and confidence. Additionally, my once pointed chest is beginning to flatten and broaden, and I'm gradually doing what I once thought was impossible for me, namely, gaining weight. Hence, for the first time in my life, I know what it is like to feel normal, to feel well, as it were.

Watching these changes unfold has been a source of great joy. Seeing, feeling, and yes, knowing that I am being transformed into a new being have given me a different image; vis-a-vis my fellow man, I no longer feel a hopeless sense of inadequacy.

Admittedly, I thought that I just couldn't live on the diet. How, I pondered, can I do without ice cream, pie, and all of the rest? But now, just as with wheezing and shortness of breath, I don't even think about it any more. In fact, I like it; the sacrifice involved gives me a sense of elevation.

You, therefore, can see that my own case history does help to justify the need for the popularity of your prospective book. To limit this discovery to the benefit of a few would be an inexcusable loss to the human race. Accordingly, I again congratulate you for undertaking your task, and wish you supreme success.

Several medical articles referred to the experiences of the late Dr. Stephen Gyland of Tampa, Florida. I wrote Dr. Gyland's widow and asked her to give me a letter with permission to use it in this publication. Her letter is as follows:

September 3, 1964

Dear Judge Blaine:

I am writing you concerning the illness and spectacular recovery of Stephen Gyland, M.D., my late husband.

In 1949, he began to have blackout spells which doctors he consulted could not account for. He had had severe tachycardia (racing heart) for several years previous to this, and went through two large northern clinics, where no reason could be found except "overwork." He was advised to give up his more taxing medical work and drink liquor to relieve the tachycardia. He did both with no help; but of course, the drinks could cause harm.

Another complaint was severe headaches, from which he had suffered for 20 years. These were diagnosed as "tension headaches," with no prescription except less work. His fatigue was great, and he woke up in the mornings more tired than when he went to bed. He was a kind, conscientious, understanding Christian general practitioner, so [he] was in great demand.

About '49 he also developed such severe arthritis in his legs and hands that he had to give up golf. Blurred and double vision plagued him and he became depressed—a complete change of personality.

He was given tests for suspected brain tumor. A 2-hour glucose tolerance test showed that his blood sugar rose to almost 280. Both he and his doctor decided that small doses of insulin might help, and they did temporarily, but he soon became almost incapacitated again. He shook like a leaf and staggered when he walked.

In 1952 our son was interning at a fine medical center and insisted that his dad should come there for more tests, which Dr. Gyland, Sr. underwent for eleven days.

At the conclusion, the neurologist said to him, "You are finished for life. You will never see another patient. You have cerebral arteriosclerosis." The medical doctor who coordinated all the work done was more gentle and said, "Come back in six months and let us see you then. You don't have diabetes, so quit taking insulin. Your future is in the hands of the Lord."

This doctor had ordered a six-hour glucose tolerance test which showed a rise to 265 and a rapid drop to 76. He said it was the "craziest curve" he had ever seen, and he advised a high protein diet with low fat. His future must have been in the hands of the Lord, as his faith had never waivered. He returned home and said, "I should be discouraged with that diagnosis—suspected cerebral arteriosclerosis—but I'm not. I have treated many patients with that, and that is not what I've got. However, that abnormal blood sugar curve interests me and I'm going to find out all I can about the opposite of diabetes."

It took a 4-month search to find out all he needed, but his recovery was very rapid when he got on the Seale Harris diet with no caffeine. Shots of . . . [trade name of calcium omitted], combined with the other treatment of diet, helped to overcome his nervousness.

His recovery was like a miracle in our lives and was the answer to fervent prayers. Later, Dr. Gyland went to see the late Seale Harris to thank him for the discovery which saved his life. He also visited Dr. E. M. Abrahamson, and was intrigued by his dedication to an illness which many doctors ignore or treat with sugar.

All of my husband's symptoms disappeared and he had seven of the happiest and most productive years of his 35 years of practice. I helped him in the office, and it was a joy to us both to see alcoholics of thirty years standing get well, to see school children who were failing recover, postpartum cases get well. One man brought his wife in and said, "This is the last chance. If you can't help her, I'm getting a divorce. She is so irritable, I can't live with her any longer." When she had been under treatment only a few weeks, he told her, "I'm falling in love with you all over again." Her disposition changed radically and her asthma disappeared. Even when they returned to their home in Michigan, the severe winter did not bring on an attack, as she told us in Christmas cards over several years.

In all, Dr. Gyland treated over 1,000 cases in his seven

years. He addressed the American Medical Association in New York City in 1957, and the Southern Medical Society in New Orleans in 1958. At the latter meeting, he showed the effect of functional hypoglycemia on skin, showing colored slides of skin conditions, before and after treatment. When the whole person was treated, the neurodermatitis got well.

Dr. Gyland's cholesterol on August 29, 1952, was 476. This was considered dangerously high at the clinic. They recommended a high protein, low fat diet. However, Dr. Gyland found the high fat diet keeps the pancreas from overactivity, and he felt that this was the more dangerous condition. So he continued to eat his two eggs a day for breakfast and to have a high protein, moderate fat diet, mostly vegetable fat. He was on no medicine to lower his cholesterol, but on October 7, 1953, it had dropped to 350, and on May 15, 1954, it was 250, and on September 22, 1955, it was 208. This was another indication that his body was functioning normally. He adhered strictly to the Seale Harris diet, plus his modification of it, and did not even take decaffeinated coffee or weak tea. Medicines often contain caffeine and their use is forbidden. He found the injections of . . . [trade name of calcium omitted] to be very beneficial. He also found that patients must be off tranquilizers for five days prior to the six-hour glucose tolerance test, since the use of tranquilizers gave a patient an abnormally high curve, a curve quite different from the curve made from the test on the patient when tranquilizers were discontinued.

His final illness followed an operation on his aorta. My present work is in the field of nutrition among the elderly, and it is challenging, too.

Sincerely,

RUTH GYLAND

I have corresponded with several allergy sufferers who informed me that they had obtained relief from injections of calcium glycerophosphate and calcium lactate. Calcium injections are reported to have been beneficial in all types of allergies, and particularly so in migraine and perennial hay fever cases.

Since I have not had any calcium injections, I can make no personal report on their effectiveness. I have found that it helps me get over a migraine attack if I make a thick mixture of nonfat powdered milk and water and eat a bowlful with a spoon, as if it were a breakfast cereal.

Another interesting letter has just reached me. It is as follows:

Oct. 5th, 1964

Dear Judge Blaine:

My sister was an asthmatic for over fifty years. Her life and death had a similarity to that of Dr. Stephen Gyland of Tampa, Florida. Both survived surgery, but failed to recover following injections of dextrose. In my sister's case the injections were given after I had informed the surgeon that she was a hypoglycemic and an asthmatic, held in complete control by a sugarless and starchless diet plus an occasional 10 cc. injection of . . . [trade name of calcium omitted] to control a low blood level serum calcium. The surgeon was also told that Dr. E. M. Abrahamson had said to me, "She will choke to death if a surgeon gives her dextrose or glucose following an operation."

She survived the surgery and was in the best of spirits even before leaving the recovery room. However, the next day her asthmatic condition had returned. Dextrose had been given. She returned home to live a miserable existence for almost eleven months. The physician who had supervised her former successful treatment for asthma never again established a control. Near the end, a specialist prescribed a derivative of cortisone. Within days she developed the "moon face" side effects. Early one morning she made one call. Death, as predicted, came a few short minutes later. . . .

J. R. Line
President, Hypoglycemia Foundation, Inc.
149 Wilmot Road
Scarsdale, N.Y.

Quite accidentally I came across a paper published in July, 1935, in *California and Western Medicine,* reporting a talk made early that year before the General Medicine Section of the California Medical Association. The subject of the paper was: "The Treatment of Asthma, with Special Reference to the Oral Use of the Adrenal Hormones and Sodium Chloride."

A letter of inquiry disclosed that the author is still living and a distinguished and active member of the California medical profession.

The remarkable thing about this paper is that it is about 15 years ahead of most other articles I have been able to find relating to the use of adrenal hormones in the treatment of allergies. I secured permission from this physician to use any or all of his 1935 article in this book. I quote from the paper:

> In August, 1932, we began feeding whole beef adrenal glands to a group of patients. . . . These were administered within a few hours from the time they were removed from the animals. Our reason for this was because of the various reports connecting this condition with adrenal deficiency.

The improvement in their energy and sense of well-being
was very definite. In September, 1932, a child whom we
were treating had been suffering from continuous asthma
for several months and was completely exhausted. With the
idea that we might at least relieve his exhaustion, we gave
him seven grams of whole raw beef adrenal gland, which
was first ground and mixed with peanut butter. That night
the child became free from asthma and remained so for
three days. This gave the impetus to the studies leading up
to the present report. Later, we began extracting the cortical
hormone. . . .

After an explanation of how the raw glands of the
animals were prepared for feeding to allergic patients, the
article continued as follows:

In nineteen children treated in the clinic and in nine adults
institutionalized, we have not failed in a single instance to
relieve the asthma. The children have almost universally
been the type who have considerable bronchitis. . . . The
cortical hormone combined with epinephrin ointment has
been quite effective in controlling eczema. . . . It seems to
be of value in migraine. . . ."

In discussing fifty cases of allergy patients treated with
cortical extract and/or epinephrin, the physician stated:

The results of all but two were satisfactory. Neither of
these patients was able to submit to a program of rest, which
is so essential to the relief of their condition, but both
patients experienced considerable increase in energy and a
feeling of increased well-being, although neither was completely freed of the attacks. . . . In speaking of relief we do
not mean temporary relief, such as is obtained from a single
injection of epinephrin, but a more permanent relief which
leaves the patient free from symptoms.

The following pages are from this 1935 medical paper:

TABLE 1.—*Results of Treatment by the Use of Adrenal Hormones Administered Orally*

Type of Patient	Type of Therapy	Improvement			Total Number Patients
		Slight	Moderate	Marked	
In-patients	Epinephrin only	0	1	1	2
Out-patients	Epinephrin only	0	2	3	5
In-patients	Cortical extract only	0	0	1	1
Out-patients	Cortical extract only	0	0	2	2
Out-patients (children)	Epinephrin and cortical extract	0	7	12	19
Out-patients (adults)	Epinephrin and cortical extract	2	2	5	9
In-patients	Epinephrin and cortical extract	0	6	4	10
	Miscellaneous therapy	0	0	2	2
		2	18	30	50

Three of adult in-patients treated less than two weeks. In each instance, relief of symptoms was obtained.

The following is typical of the type of children that we have been treating:

Case No. C-10434.—Male, aged eight years. Suffering from severe asthma. Treated with cortical extract and epinephrin orally, and a diet giving acid ash.

At the age of three years the patient suddenly developed asthma. He was given potassium iodide, ephedrin, lactose, Maltine, and cod-liver oil, with no appreciable effect. In the spring of 1932 he was found sensitive to 57 of 300 antigens. He was given treatment without relief. In 1933 his asthma became worse, and in December was extremely distressing. His attacks were usually preceded by colds and were accompanied by severe coughing and wheezing. The attacks were milder during the summer and more severe during the winter. He gave a history of having little energy and always complained of being tired.

Examination revealed a red-haired, pale-skinned child of the angiospastic pseudo-anemic type. He had hypertrophied tonsils and enlargement of the cervical lymph glands. His chest showed many rhonchi and râles throughout, and was markedly emphysematous. The x-ray showed increased linear markings radiating from the hilum, suggestive of chronic bronchitis. Calcified nodes were present within the hilum on both sides.

A diagnosis of chronic asthma, with bronchitis, was made.

Although the patient had several colds, after treatment was begun they were less intense. After treatment began, February 10, 1934, he did not have a single paroxysm of asthma. During the first half of the school year, 1933-1934, he had missed school nearly half of the time, on account of colds and asthma. During the second half he lost only two weeks, and during the year of 1934-1935, he did not lose a single day of schooling. Previously he was unable to play with other children; but now he is interested in athletics and is a leader in sports, and it is with the greatest difficulty that he is kept from playing too hard. Severe physical exertion brings on coughing spells. During the eighteen months under treatment he has gained fourteen pounds, and his physical condition is excellent.

The use of ground adrenals prior to 1935 for relief of allergies reminds me of the use of ground liver in the 1920's, when liver was found to be a cure for the then-fatal pernicious anemia, also known as Addison's anemia.

As I studied this remarkable report made many years ago, I was thankful that I did not have to swallow a ground-up mixture of raw beef adrenal gland and peanut butter to be cured of my allergies. Apparently, in 1935 little was known about the high protein, low carbohydrate diet now being used with adrenal cortex extract in the treatment of allergy cases.

Last fall a grandmother serving on one of our county jury panels told me her daughter was having a lot of difficulty with the milk formulas for her baby. She said the baby's face had been covered with some kind of rash almost since birth, even though the doctor had made several changes in the baby's diet.

I suggested to the juror that she have her daughter ask the doctor about putting the infant on a low carbohydrate (no sugar), high protein diet and see if that would clear up the skin condition. The report came to me some weeks later that when my suggestion was communicated to the doctor, he became furious and stated that he wished judges and lawyers would stop trying to practice medicine. He told the baby's mother that a rabbit's foot tied around her child's neck would do as much good as what I had recommended.

Without the doctor's knowledge or consent, the mother went ahead with a sugarless, low carbohydrate, high protein diet, and, in a week or ten days, the infant's skin cleared. Later the doctor called me and said two other mothers had gotten rid of skin eruptions on their babies' faces with what he called "your diet." He asked, "What is this, and where did you get onto it?" I had to be in court in his town in a few days, so I brought him all of the medical material I had on hypoadrenocorticism.

Months later, this doctor told me that whenever an infant had any allergic manifestations, including colic or spitting up food, he put the baby on the low carbohydrate, high protein diet and prescribed adrenal cortex tablets. He said this routine had worked in every case in which it had been tried.

When the doctor returned the medical papers I had given him, I observed he gave me two or three additional medical articles on allergies. One of them was of particular interest to me since it contained medical information about steroid (cortisone) therapy which other doctors had not given me. It stated that intensive, long-term cortisone therapy can damage the adrenals to the degree that sometimes neither medication nor diet are effective, and that an intensive steroid (cortisone) therapy for only a month or so often caused patients on the low carbodydrate, high protein diet and adrenal cortex medication to respond much more slowly than did those who had received no steroids.

Since the treatment discussed in the preceding chapters can be used effectively for allergics of all ages, the future of the allergic child is much brighter than it has been in the past. An allergic child is usually an unhappy child. The parents and the child have emotional problems they can't solve and which make the allergies worse.

In the divorce courts, I have talked with scores of small allergic children (usually asthmatics), who actually had feelings of guilt over their parents' marriage breakups.

It is not difficult to understand why a child has such a guilt complex when a mother says, in the presence of her children, "Then to add to all of my troubles, Jane started having asthmatic attacks." It never once occurred to this self-pitying mother that the parents' actions and conduct could produce enough emotional trauma to make any small, susceptible child asthmatic.

Many doctors tell parents of allergic children to treat their sons and daughters as if they were normal and healthy children. That, however, is frequently impossible, for if an allergic child is sent outdoors to play in the snow with the same amount of clothing worn by other children, the chances are he will get bronchitis or pneumonia. If he gets some kind of infection, even an ordinary cold, in the fall, he sometimes will have difficulty getting over it all winter.

When parents understand how important it is that allergic children suffer no unnecessary emotional upsets, and that children can be cured of allergies by diet and medication, much of childhood's unhappiness will be prevented. Since the psychologists tell us the unhappy child will be the unhappy adult, it is imperative that our allergic children be cured of their allergies while they are still young. I know from experience the tragedy of being a sickly child. I never heard of the word "allergy" until I was grown. In my childhood there was little that could be done for allergies except to try to make the best of a bad situation. Thank God, children are now living in the age of medical miracles.

Speaking in the language of my profession, the law, this new method of treating and curing allergic sufferers needs no advocates to plead its cause before the tribunals of modern medicine. It is entitled to impartial, unbiased, and fair hearings before the supreme court of medicine— the physicians of the nation. Whenever and wherever it has been fairly, honestly, and competently tested by doctors, the results have been so much better than were anticipated that it has already been proven to be a miracle of modern medicine.

APPENDIX A

*Classification and Composition of Certain Foods
as to Carbohydrate, Protein, and Fat Content**

VEGETABLES

3 PER CENT CARBOHYDRATE AVERAGE

Asparagus
Beans, green or wax
Broccoli
Brussels sprouts
Cabbage
Cabbage, Chinese
Cauliflower
Celery
Chard or Swiss chard
Collards
Cucumbers
Eggplant
Endive
Escarole
Greens, beet, dandelion, mustard or turnip greens
Kale or sea kale
Leeks
Lettuce
Okra
Olives, ripe or green
Onions, cooked
Peppers, green or red
Pickles, unsweetened, dill or sour
Radishes
Rhubarb
Sauerkraut
Spinach
Summer squash or cymlings
Tomatoes or tomato juice
Water cress

6 PER CENT CARBOHYDRATE AVERAGE

Artichokes, globe or French
Beets
Carrots
Kohlrabi
Onions, raw

* From Yater's *Fundamentals of Internal Medicine*, Fourth Edition, 1954, with permission from Appleton-Century-Crofts.

Oyster plant or salsify
Pumpkin
Rutabagas
Squash, winter or Hubbard
Turnips, white or yellow

15 Per Cent Carbohydrate Average

Artichokes, Jerusalem
Green peas
Parsnips

20 Per Cent Carbohydrate Average

Corn
Hominy, cooked
Lima beans, canned
Macaroni, boiled
Noodles, cooked
Potato
Rice, boiled
Shelled beans, cooked
Spaghetti, cooked

FRUITS

5 Per Cent Carbohydrate Average (canned without sugar)

Apricots
Blackberries
Cherries, red or white
Loganberries

Peaches
Raspberries
Rhubarb, fresh
Strawberries

10 Per Cent Carbohydrate Average

Blackberries, fresh
Cantaloupe, muskmelon, honeydew, Spanish melon
Cranberries
Gooseberries
Grapefruit or grapefruit juice
Lemons
Oranges or orange juice
Peaches, fresh
Pears, alligator or avocado
Pineapple, fresh
Strawberries, fresh
Tangerines or tangelos
Watermelon

15 Per Cent Carbohydrate Average

Apples
Apricots, fresh
Blueberries or huckleberries
Cherries, sour
Currants
Loganberries, fresh
Nectarines
Pears
Raspberries, red or black, fresh

20 Per Cent Carbohydrate Average

Bananas
Grapes or grape juice
Plums
Prunes

COMPOSITION OF VARIOUS FOODS

Average Composition of 100 Grams

	Carbohydrate Grams	Protein Grams	Fat Grams
VEGETABLES AND FRUITS:			
3 per cent vegetables	3	1	0
6 per cent vegetables	6	1	0
15 per cent vegetables	15	2	0
20 per cent vegetables:			
Potato	20	2	0
Shelled beans	20	7	0
Green corn	20	3	1
5 per cent fruits	5	1	0
10 per cent fruits	10	1	0
15 per cent fruits	15	1	0
20 per cent fruits	20	2	0
Green olives	2	1	10
Ripe olives	4	1	20
CEREALS AND BREADSTUFFS:			
Breakfast cereals, dry	80	10	5
Breakfast cereals, cooked	11	1	0
White bread	53	9	2
Whole wheat bread	49	10	1
Rye bread	53	9	1
Wheat flour	76	8	1
Soda crackers	73	10	9
Soy beans	8	38	15
DAIRY PRODUCTS:			
Whole milk	5	3	4
Skimmed milk	5	3	1
Cream, 20 per cent fat	5	3	20
Cream, 30 per cent fat	4	3	30
Cream, 40 per cent fat	3	2	40
Buttermilk	5	3	1
Cheese	0	29	36
Cottage cheese	4	21	1

Eggs, each	0	6	6
Egg white (one)	0	3	0
Egg yolk (one)	0	3	6
MEATS AND FISH:			
Meat, cooked	0	25	15
Fat meat, cooked	0	25	30
Fish (halibut, lake trout, perch, white fish)	0	18	5
Salmon, fresh or canned	0	22	13
Oysters	4	6	1
Liver	2	20	3
Fat bacon	0	10	67
Lean bacon	0	16	43
Cooked bacon	0	25	50
FATS:			
Butter	0	0	85
Lard tallow, oleomargarine, crisco, bacon fat	0	0	85-100
Olive oil and other oils	0	0	100
Mayonnaise (see below)	0	0	85
Peanut butter	6	29	46
NUTS:			
Butternuts	3	28	61
Brazil nuts	7	17	67
Hickory nuts	11	15	67
Black walnuts	12	28	56
Pecans	13	11	71
Filberts	13	16	65
Beechnuts	13	22	57
English walnuts	16	17	63
Almonds	3	21	55
Peanuts	6	30	50
Chestnuts	42	6	5

APPENDIX B

A valuable publication on the nutritive value of foods, the yield of cooked meat per pound of raw meat, and the recommended daily dietary allowances is *Home and Garden Bulletin, No. 72,* United States Department of Agriculture, issued September, 1960, and prepared by the Institute of Home Economics, Agricultural Research Service. This bulletin, about thirty pages in length, is revised from time to time in accordance with newer knowledge of nutritional needs and is often available in county home demonstration offices. Other publications by the National Academy of Sciences, National Research Council, Washington 25, D.C., are usually available in public libraries or may be purchased at modest prices.

Charts and booklets showing the proper weights for men and women of various ages and builds and the significance and prevention of obesity may be had on request and without cost from most major life insurance companies or their agents.